THE HUMAN BRAIN

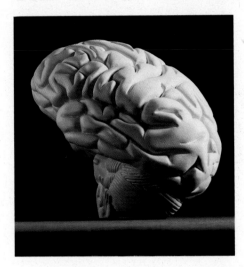

AUDITORY STIMULATION

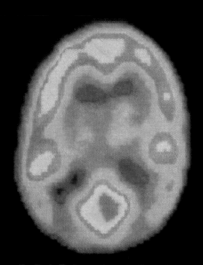

RESTING STATE

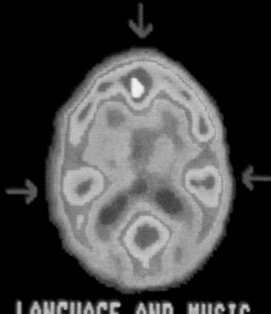

LANGUAGE AND MUSIC

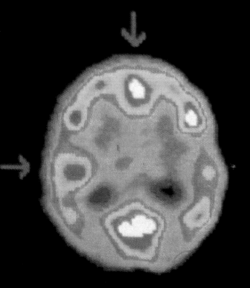

LANGUAGE

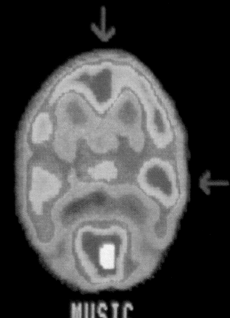

MUSIC

THE HUMAN BRAIN

DICK GILLING AND
ROBIN BRIGHTWELL

Facts On File Publications
460 Park Avenue South
New York, N.Y. 10016

BY ARRANGEMENT WITH ORBIS PUBLISHING LTD.,
LONDON

DEDICATION
To those whose handicaps and disabilities have helped towards the
understanding of the healthy human brain.

HALF-TITLE PAGE
The human brain: increasingly the symbol of scientific controversy and
daring investigation.

FRONTISPIECE
A PET scan of a living human brain. Areas which are most active are
shown in red, and in these examples it can be seen that listening to
language causes the left side of the brain to show activity, while listening
to music causes more activity on the right side. Even at rest, the brain
remains active in some areas.

First published in the United States by
Facts On File, Inc.
460 Park Avenue South
New York, N.Y. 10016

First published 1982 by Orbis Publishing Limited, London

© 1982 Dick Gilling and Robin Brightwell

Library of Congress Cataloging in Publication Data

Gilling, Dick.
  The human brain.

  Bibliography: p.
  Includes index.
  1. Brain.   I. Brightwell, Robin.   II. Title.
QP376.G5 1983   612'.82   82-15467
  ISBN 0-87196-710-3

Printed in Great Britain
10 9 8 7 6 5 4 3 2 1

CONTENTS

Authors' Acknowledgments

Soon after we started research for the television series on which this book is based, we agreed that it would be futile even to attempt to deal with all the science of the brain. This could not be done in seventy programmes, much less in seven, and so this book is not an encyclopaedia of the brain. But we have added a short Atlas of the Brain to which the reader can refer for clarification of words or terms used in the rest of the text, and which gives a simple account of how the brain is put together, and how it works. There are very many schools of thought in the field, and we have tried to reflect all of them as fairly as we can, but in the process many details have been omitted to give an overall view.

During the two years that it has taken to make our programmes, we have relied with our colleagues, on the goodwill and the advice of over a hundred scientists in all fields, in Europe, Britain, and the United States. It is their information that we have used in constructing the programmes and in writing this book; our effort has been to combine that information in a comprehensible way, and to simplify without, we hope, misleading. These scientists have given us their time generously, have answered (often stupid) questions courteously, and have in many cases subjected themselves to the stress and indignity of being filmed. Only a few could be included in the programmes; but many others helped to construct the series by their advice, or pointed us in new directions. Without the generosity of all these people in the scientific community our work would have been impossible, and we owe them a great debt of gratitude. With their help, we have been guided on a voyage of discovery, the results of which are contained in this book; and in many happy memories.

Even the most apparently iron-bound results of these scientists may be subject to different interpretations; science progresses by disproving theories as well as by proving them. Inevitably, we have sometimes been arrogant enough to give opinions, or theories, as well as facts. We hope that they are well-founded.

It would also have been impossible to make the programmes or write this book without the collaboration of the many patients who generously agreed to be filmed. A person who is in some way handicapped, who cannot speak clearly, whose memory is grossly defective, or who has spent many years in psychiatric hospitals, is easily hurt. Many people shared their pains and frustrations with us, and allowed us to watch them and film them in conditions that throw a revealing and potentially cruel light on their handicap. Like us, they were convinced that meeting a problem face to face may not be the easiest way to live; but it gives understanding where that is most needed. Most of these brave people will never be cured, but they taught us that they were not cases, or examples, but always people, like those of us lucky enough not to be maimed by injury or disease. They gave us perhaps the most important information of all: the brain is not so sacred that an injury to it takes away our humanity. To all of them we are deeply grateful.

A television programme is a collective enterprise. We are also in the debt of all those who worked on these programmes, not only for their professional skills and advice, but because their questions and conversation obliged us to re-work and clarify our ideas, and led us into paths we might have otherwise missed. Our thanks are due also to the BBC, and to Belgian Radio and Television and the Australian Broadcasting Commission, who provided the finance and encouragement to produce the programmes.

We would also like to thank the researchers, Gill Nevill and Max Whitby; the picture researcher, Pamela Smith; the production assistants, Ann Larman and Jane Amin; the film cameramen, Colin Munn and Ian Stone; the assistant cameramen, Richard Adam and John Rhodes; the sound recordist, Alan Cooper; the film editors, Les Newman, Paul Pierrot, David Lee and Michael Flynn; the assistant film editors, David Good, Christy Hanna and Nick Morris; the graphic designer, Darrell Pocket; the visual effects designer, Mat Irvine, and the many other artists and technicians who contributed to the series.

Introduction

As infants grow through their first years of life they gradually develop an identity. Each child gets the feeling that he or she is a unique human being. It is that feeling, remaining with the individual until death, which makes it difficult for us humans to comprehend the contributions of our brains to ourselves.

To imagine how the firing of nerve cells in the brain and limbs can move an arm or leg is easy enough. But to accept that nerve cells and nerve cells alone are responsible for language, memory, imagination, and feeling of identity, the self, in fact the mind as a whole, is not easy and for most individuals has until now been impossible. How could the feeling of oneself arise from millions and millions of electrical signals in the brain? The complexity and actual perception of one's own feelings make this 'mechanistic' approach to the human being unacceptable to most individuals. Religion, particularly Christianity, argues that there is a soul, separate from the brain, even from the mind. Even those who are not believers often feel that to explain human function through the electrical and chemical signals of the brain is to convert man into nothing more than a machine.

In this one book we cannot hope, nor would we wish, to counter the arguments of religion, or to argue against the *feeling* that individuality must be more than the product of the firing of nerve cells, but we do wish to allay fears that this approach turns humans into nothing more than machines.

Allaying those fears was relatively easy in the actual programmes on which this book is based, since we could film those people whose brains and minds we were describing and show, merely by their behaviour and what they said, that they were humans, whatever mechanistic explanations we gave for their activities or disabilities. In a book it is more difficult to give that impression.

The individual is made up of the human faculties which depend entirely upon the firing of his or her nerve cells (and all the other cells in the body and brain). But the whole individual is far more than the mere sum of all his or her nerve cells parts. Human beings are often credited with a separate mind that is of a different nature from the nerve cells of the brain; the underlying and powerful reasons why the mind is so often seen in that light, as separate, are either failure of imagination, or of courage, or both, on the part of scientist, philosopher or plain ordinary person. Imagination is needed to see how nerve cells can give rise to the wildest dreams, greatest achievements, and worst excesses of man; courage is needed to be prepared to lay the human a little barer, metaphorically more naked, than he usually wishes to be. The idea that we arise from no more than electrical and chemical signals may create a lonely feeling, but not if one takes the wonderfully optimistic and natural human view that we are more than the sum of those parts. We still have choices, free-will. We still have moral values. We still have love and imagination. We still appreciate beauty. The modern, mechanistic approach does not make man into a laboratory rat, but it raises a fascinating question: if biological elements alone give rise to all that is human, how on earth do they actually achieve it?

We have used the mechanistic approach throughout this book because we believe science is just on the verge of throwing light on this question, far though we still are from a complete answer. In each of our chapters we have attempted to give some insight into the brain's control of such faculties, but in none of them are humans de-humanized. We hope this insight makes them marginally more aware of what might be going on inside their heads and possibly a little prouder of it.

An Atlas of the Brain

This brief, illustrated account of the parts of the human brain and their connections will make the following chapters easier to read. Some of its information may recur later, often in more detail, where it is of importance to the topic of a particular chapter.

INSIDE THE SKULL

The brain of a human being, when exposed, looks rather like an enormous walnut; it weighs about three or three and a half pounds and is made up, like other organs, of cells. Unlike a walnut, it has been mapped in minute detail; even the apparently random surface corrugations by which we all recognize the brain have names. Since the learned men who first dissected the brain used Latin and Greek, the languages of scholars over the centuries, the names of various parts of the brain are based on Latin and Greek terminology, which may at first be alarming; but one soon realizes it only represents a series of valiant attempts at describing the indescribable. So, that wrinkled outside of the *cerebrum* (brain) is the *cortex* (bark) and is divided into *gyri* (ridges) and *sulci* (valleys). The small, ridged projection at the back is the *cerebellum* (little brain), and so on.

THE CEREBRAL HEMISPHERES

The wrinkled cortex is the surface layer, about 3 or 4 mm thick, of the two most notable parts of the human brain, the cerebral hemispheres, which are far larger in the human than in any other animal. As a result of the wrinkling of the cortex, the area of cortex is much greater than that of the skull in which it is contained. The two cerebral hemispheres, almost but not quite mirror images of one another, together constitute the cerebrum; and each hemisphere is divided into lobes, the 'continents' of the cerebrum. At the front, of course, the frontal lobe; at the side, the temporal lobe; on top, the parietal lobe; and at the back of the head, the occipital lobe. Each lobe is roughly associated with a different function: the parietal lobes seem to contain areas responsible for co-ordinating the input of our sense organs and the output of instructions to our muscles;

VIEW FROM THE TOP
The wrinkled surface of the two cerebral hemispheres, the cortex, much greater in area than the cortex of any comparable animal brain.

Right hemisphere

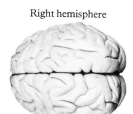

Left hemisphere

LOBES OF THE BRAIN
The frontal lobe (*left*) under the forehead, may deal with matters of the intellect, including planning; the parietal lobes (*top*) include sensory and motor areas; the temporal lobes (*centre*) include regions concerned with memory and emotion; the occipital lobe (*right*) includes visual regions.

Frontal lobe   Parietal lobe

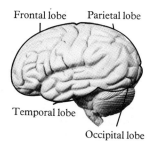

Temporal lobe

Occipital lobe

and the temporal and frontal lobes seem to dea [...]
matters, such as speech and memory.

The two hemispheres are joined by a thick [...]
fibres, the *corpus callosum* (or tough body). Bor [...]
callosum is the *limbic* (bordering) lobe, an area i[...]
other things, emotion. Then comes the egg-shaped *thalamus* (inner
chamber, or bedroom!) which is junction and interchange for many
fibres, almost in the centre of the brain; below it, the *hypothalamus*
(below the thalamus), concerned with emotions and regulation of
body temperature and state, and with the secretions of the pituitary
gland, nestling in a bony hollow at the base of the skull. All these
structures, with many subdivisions, constitute the forebrain.

THE LEFT HEMISPHERE

This hemisphere, in the great
majority of cases, is responsible for
language. It also contains regions
responsible for vision, sense and
movement on the right side of the
body.

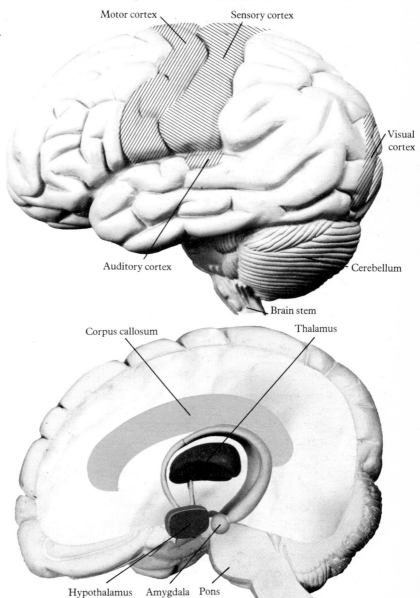

Motor cortex   Sensory cortex

Visual
cortex

Auditory cortex   Cerebellum

Brain stem

Corpus callosum   Thalamus

INSIDE THE RIGHT HEMISPHERE

The connection between the
hemispheres is the corpus
callosum. The thalamus and
hypothalamus both contain many
nuclei dealing with specific
functions of body and brain.

Hypothalamus   Amygdala   Pons

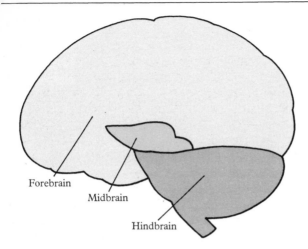

Forebrain

Midbrain

Hindbrain

THE BRAIN HIERARCHY
The brain stem, of hind and mid-brain, evolved earlier than the forebrain, which is more associated with so-called higher mental functions or conscious states.

The midbrain (or *mesencephalon*) is much smaller; among its duties are the control of responses to sight and sound, and some control of sleep and waking. The hindbrain includes the cerebellum, involved in the management of movement, and many tiny bumps and lumps with particular functions, too numerous to name. Midbrain and hindbrain are often grouped together, and called the brain stem, one of the few instantly intelligible terms in the neurosciences.

FROM BRAIN TO BODY

Connecting the brain stem to the rest of the body, the spinal cord contains regions which have their own functions; NCOs, perhaps, to the brain's officer-class. But much of its bulk carries fibres running from the brain to connect with muscles or sense organs far away from the brain, in fingertips or feet.

The brain, the brain stem and the spinal cord together are the central nervous system. The network running through the rest of our bodies, nerves telling us about toothache or biting fleas, is the peripheral nervous system. But beware of placing them in separate compartments; the peripheral nerves are constantly supplying the brain with information to update its plans, and the brain is constantly altering the receptivity of the peripheral nerves; there is a continuous dialogue between all parts of the brain and the rest of the nervous system. Our plan of lobes and Latin names does not divide the brain into separate compartments. The job of being human is shared among all of them, and the labels were attached only by fallible mortals trying to map a jungle.

There are many more parts of the brain, large and small, that have been identified and given names; too many to include in this survey. We have avoided the use of these technical terms as much as possible in the following chapters, but where their use is unavoidable, reference to the Glossary should help.

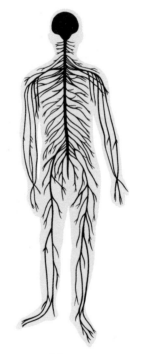

THE NERVE NETWORK
From the central nervous system of brain and spinal cord, peripheral nerves spread to each part of the body. The illustration shows only the main nerve trunks, from which other tiny nerves branch.

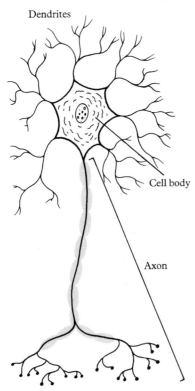

Dendrites

Cell body

Axon

THE NERVE CELL

All the nerve cells, or neurones, in the system have this general plan: from the cell body sprout dendrites, to receive impulses; and an axon, to send impulses.

THE NERVOUS SYSTEM ANALYSED

The whole of the nervous system is made up of cells. Nerve cells (or neurones; neurons in the United States), unlike other cells in the human body (blood cells, for example), send out many fibres or processes. Some, the dendrites, receive signals from other cells; others, the axons, which usually also branch, are the message senders; they may be as short as a tenth of a millimetre, or as much as a metre long. Each nerve cell or neurone is in contact with about 1000 other nerve cells. And the brain itself is made up of about 1,000,000,000,000 nerve cells; maybe ten times more or ten times less. The number is too big to comprehend: but, if you spent one second counting each nerve cell, you would be at it for 30,000 years or so; to count each contact, multiply by another few thousand, for nerve cells usually have more than one point of contact with each other. The grey matter of the brain, including the outer 3 or 4 mm of the cortex, and various other areas, is composed of the cell bodies; the white matter is composed of axons, coated with insulating sheaths of fat.

A cell passes information along its fibres in the form of electrical signals (varying not in strength but in frequency – a sequence of dots, fast or slow), but the message passes to the next cell, at a synapse, in chemical form. The *synapse* (handclasp) is the microscopic area in which messages pass from one cell to another. When the electric wave reaches the synapse, it causes the cell to release a chemical substance which diffuses across the synaptic gap to the next cell, which then converts the chemical message once again to electricity. Once used, the chemical is reabsorbed into the cell or destroyed by an enzyme.

Each nerve cell has thousands of synapses. The synapses, converging on a cell, determine democratically how the cell will act. Some, the excitatory synapses, will cause the cell to fire, while others, the inhibitory synapses, will prevent it firing. So rather roughly, if more excitatory than inhibitory synapses act, the cell will vote to fire; more inhibitory, and it will refuse to fire. And, since the synapses monitor the 'votes' of other nerve cells, the democracy is an all-embracing one.

In all likelihood, the position of synapses also determines the strength of their influence; synapses on the dendrites may be less powerful than those on the cell body, or vice versa. Different types of cell, and there are many, may process the 'vote' in different ways, but we do not yet know how. It is just possible that cell A may have an inhibitory effect on cell B but an excitatory effect on cell C; even the rule about chemical transmission is not inviolable; just after chemical synaptic action was established, in the 1950s, some electrical synapses were discovered. There are even axon-to-axon and dendrite-to-dendrite synapses, which deepen the puzzle still more. In short, the brain is full of surprises, and it seems to be the case that no simple rules will necessarily be obeyed in all circumstances.

THE CHEMICAL HANDSHAKE

The chemistry of the brain, too, has turned out to be less straightforward and far more exciting than we dreamed of, even ten years ago. At that time, the general consensus was that only two chemicals, or two classes of chemicals, would be involved in synaptic transmission: one would be inhibitory, one excitatory. They were named neuro-transmitters; and it was held that each cell would produce and use only one, either inhibitory or excitatory. This dogma is no longer universally accepted. Furthermore, many more possible neuro-transmitters have been discovered; currently over thirty candidates exist. Each of these chemicals may well have different and complex pathways in the brain, augmenting or modulating the pathways that connect cells or regions we already know. And they may not act in the classical fashion of the neuro-transmitter. It seems possible that they may modulate the effects of the cell-to-cell transmission in some way by affecting the inner chemistry of the cell, and therefore its electrical properties.

This area of research is the most rapidly expanding of all, and without doubt new discoveries will add to, and alter, our present conception of the brain.

All of this complexity, however, can be made to conform, more or less, to a simple theory of what the brain does. Inputs from our sense organs, eyes, ears and so on, enter the brain, which decodes and processes them, and sends output to our muscles, resulting in actions. The only hitch is that we, as yet, know much less about processing than we do about input or output. Even so, we do know that some of the processes are born into us; hard-wired, as some neuro-scientists call it. Others seem to be learned, which suggests that not all the brain is hard-wired, but that its connections can be broken and reconnected in different ways.

Nerve cells in the brain die from about the time when we are eighteen, and new ones do not grow; but existing cells can put out new fibres, and send them long distances. This is easier for peripheral nerves than for nerve cells in the central nervous system, but even there it is not impossible. It may be that we can manage with fewer brain cells than we are born with; but we would be rash to surrender any of them without a struggle. The brain probably manages to cope with the death of cells, either through age or injury, by making new connections; but even for the hundreds of millions of cells in the brain, there has to be an end to this process somewhere.

In some ways, the central nervous system is cut off from the rest of the body. The so-called 'blood-brain barrier' serves to prevent many potentially unwelcome substances in the blood from

NERVE FIBRES
At a magnification of 5000 times, mushroom-shaped swellings containing synapses are visible at the axon tips.

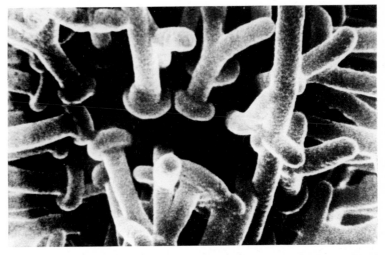

reaching the brain, presumably by a filtering process of some kind in the blood-vessels supplying the brain. The brain and spinal cord have their own fluid supply in the cerebro-spinal fluid that surrounds them and fills their cavities; but they have a blood supply, too. In fact, though the brain is only two per cent of the whole body's weight, it consumes twenty per cent of the oxygen and glucose carried by the blood – ten times more than its share. If the blood supply is interrupted for more than a couple of minutes or so, the cells are so starved (they carry no reserves) that they will die. That is what happens to part of the brain in a stroke.

It is one thing to describe the brain in terms of a simple atlas, as we have done here, or even in more detailed form, analogous to an Ordnance Survey map. (That the latter can now be done is a tribute to the industry and skill of brain anatomists, whose work continues to illuminate our picture of the structure of the brain.) It is another thing to relate this structure to the functions of its various elements, and then to relate those functions to our own behaviour.

But we can already take some infant steps along that road, and begin to see how the brain gives us our ability to speak, see, move or remember. The following seven chapters describe some of the ways in which we are beginning to understand how the brain may accomplish its formidable tasks. If we begin to understand how we act, some day we may understand also why we act as we do, come to terms with ourselves, and solve the problems that have pursued the human race ever since Cain killed Abel, or since Pandora opened her box, or even since Prometheus stole fire. We had better start somewhere.

CHAPTER 1

MEMORY

It is not always possible to understand a machine by analysing its parts. We need to know what the machine is intended to do. There is no doubt that we use our brains for remembering, but before we try to track down memory in our brain cells, we must know the nature of the process of remembering. That is the business of the psychologist. Later in this chapter we shall see that we can begin to trace some connections between our memories and our brains in physical terms, but there is first of all much to reveal about our understanding of memory.

Memory takes many forms. It is the short-term memory which enables us to remember a telephone number, for example, just long enough for us to dial it. Once the number is ringing then we forget it. That memory needs to last only seconds. But what most of us mean by memory is what is called by psychologists 'long-term memory'.

Typically our long-term memories are our recollections of childhood, or of the events of last Christmas, and naturally their durability and vividness will inevitably vary from one person to the next, and according to circumstances.

There are also different categories of memories stored in the brain. We certainly have recollections stored variously in the form of words and pictures, but we can also recall sounds, smells and tastes from our memory store. Add to these the ability quickly to recover unpractised physical skills, like icing a cake or riding a bicycle, and the brain's memory function begins to look very impressive.

Perhaps impressive is the key word. For however else our memories differ, they have made sufficient impression upon us all to qualify for storage, then to be stored and, sometimes, to qualify for recall when we most need them.

In this chapter we shall investigate the nature of the process of remembering. We shall see that we can begin to trace some connections between our memories and our brains in physical terms. And by looking at the way in which memories disappear, the ways in which we forget, we shall gain a greater understanding of memory.

REMEMBRANCE OF TIMES PAST

We visited the late actor and comedian, Stanley Holloway, who had celebrated his ninetieth birthday. Stanley Holloway's mind was active and alert, and he seemed a great deal younger than his advanced years. We asked him what he could remember of his early childhood.

> My earliest memory? It goes way back. I think I was about three or just over. I was down at the seaside with my parents and paddling along at the edge of the water. And it came to a breakwater, and on the side where I was paddling it was just over my ankles, but I stepped over the breakwater and there was about six to eight feet of water the other side because it went right down, and I stepped right over into it. And I do remember distinctly not being able to breathe. My face was down in the water, and the next thing I remember was my mother drying me out in the digs where we were staying, and my father getting his clothes off because he'd gone into the water after me. That's my earliest recollection.

It is evident that Stanley Holloway had a very retentive memory. There are about ten factual recollections in his description of his earliest memory. But he was himself very aware of the problems of being ninety: 'Oh, actually it's things I did fifty years ago I find I can remember – but things I did five weeks ago? I have no idea.'

We reminded him of a film he made in the 1940s with Tommy Trinder, *Champagne Charlie*. Stanley thought about it for a moment and then said, 'Yes, I remember all those drinks. We had a number of drinks – burgundy, claret and port and, er. . . .' He began to sing. 'I like a glass of sherry wine, a glass of sherry wine, for when I'm drinking sherry, I'm so awfully awfully merry. Oh, a glass of sherry wine . . . la, la . . . something like that.' He paused and looked a little apologetic. 'I've forgot it now,' he said.

Anecdotal evidence such as that gathered from the grand old man of the stage has to be viewed with caution, but there is a good deal that suggests that the longer memories are actually retained the stronger they become, and the less liable to disruption, in other words to forgetting. Conversely, it seems that early stages of memory can easily be disrupted.

We shall go on to look at the ways in which psychologists of different eras have attempted controlled tests on the process of storing information in the brain.

LEARNING BY REPETITION

Psychologists today are concerned that their tests and their theories should relate to the real world. That has not always been the case.

baf	schük
dak	jöm
fek	bät
gel	büp
kim	dit
jin	don
kip	fol
lor	güm
mun	hep
num	jaun
pät	kes
rösch	lop
söt	lim
teit	pep
wauch	rak

Time in seconds to re-learn words after 24 hours
1200 · 1000 · 800 · 600 · 400 · 200

Number of repetitions on day 1
0 8 16 24 32 42 53 64

LEARNING PARROT-FASHION
Ebbinghaus's proof that successful repetitions on day 1 lead to better retention on day 2 even when the subject learns nonsense words. The data used in this chart is taken from Ebbinghaus's book, *Memory*, published in New York in 1913.

Hermann Ebbinghaus, the father of the psychological study of memory, was anxious to exclude the real world from his experiments, and his legacy to the study of psychology may therefore in some ways have been a negative one.

Ebbinghaus made his great study while he was still a comparatively young man in the early 1880s. He meticulously drew up a series of lists of nonsense words, each consisting of a vowel with a consonant on either side, and rigorously excluded anything that might contain any meaning for him. The task he set himself, and it was an epic one, was to memorize sequences of hundreds of the words. He consistently tested himself at the same time on each day, and he excluded all outside influences. In other words he reduced the conditions of learning to the simplest (and arguably the least realistic) possible.

Ebbinghaus repeated the syllables over to himself at the rate of 150 a minute until he had learnt each group perfectly. He would then re-learn the same group the next day at the same time until he had once again acquired perfect retention. Ebbinghaus discovered that he learned at a constant rate. The more often he repeated the syllables to himself the better they stuck, it was as simple as that. But his discovery will come as no surprise to those who advocate learning multiplication tables by rote. Rather understandably, after two years of such exacting experiments, Ebbinghaus left the study of memory. He produced much data but no theories. Yet Ebbinghaus showed that even so complex a subject as memory could be focused sharply by reducing it to a simple model.

CONTEXT-RELATED LEARNING

Alan Baddeley is Director of the Medical Research Council's Applied Psychology Unit at Cambridge. When he was at Stirling University he was responsible for one of the more spectacular

NERVE FIBRES AND CELLS IN THE CEREBELLUM
The deeply folded structure of the cortex can be clearly seen in these illustrations (*see An Atlas of the Brain on page 10*). In the silver-stained section (*above*) the fibres, mostly dendrites, show up as dark threads. The cell bodies are in the golden-yellow area. In the section (*below*) the cell bodies are stained in the dark red colour, and the fibres are pale.

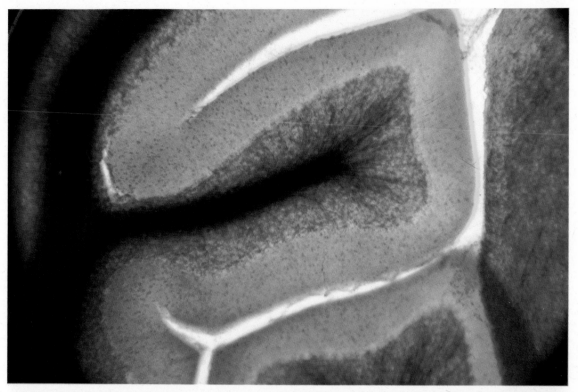

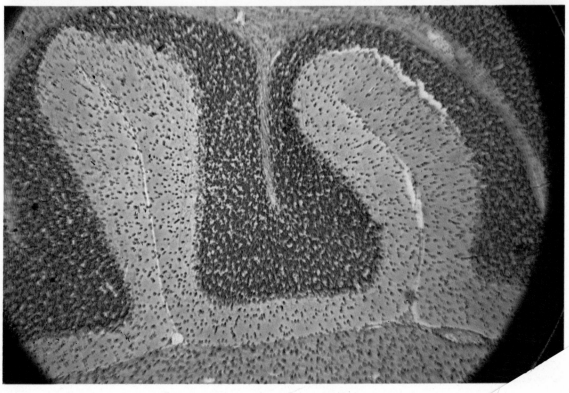

83-1959

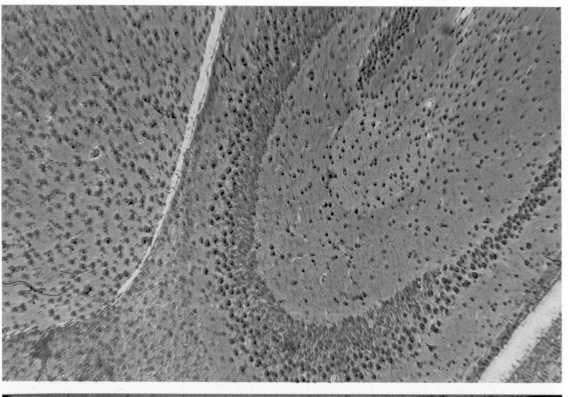

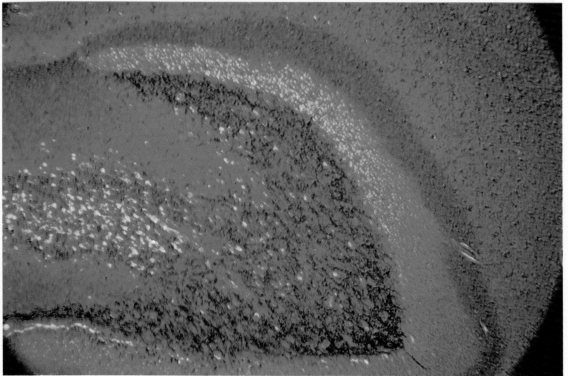

CELLS CONNECTED WITH MEMORY

This illustration (*above left*) shows two types of cell in the part of the brain associated with memory function. The hippocampus is so named because in some sections it resembles the sea horse in shape.

CELLS THAT GROW NEW SYNAPSES

In this toothlike area of the hippocampus (*below left*), the regular layers of cells are clearly seen. This regularity makes it possible to use the 'slice' technique employed in brain experiments.

EXPERIMENTS UNDERWATER

1 A Learning words underwater
  B Return to surface
  C Recalling words underwater
2 A Learning new words underwater
  B Return to surface
  C Recalling words on surface
Repeated trials showed words learned and recalled in the same context were retained better.

experiments in the psychology of memory. He persuaded six subjects to learn lists of words while they were under water, and then compared their recall of the words under water with their recall of a second list learned under water but recalled on dry land. Words both learned and recalled under water were dramatically better remembered than words learned and recalled in different environments. It seems, too, that what we learn when drunk we remember better drunk than sober. Less remarkable, however, are the results of studying for an examination in the room in which the examination is to take place.

Baddeley's underwater experiment shows that the context, or the environment, in which we learn can have a powerful effect on our ability to recall. The context presumably provides clues which enable us to code information more completely for subsequent retrieval from the file. But the experiment also suggests that when normal people forget, the faulty component is recall, not the

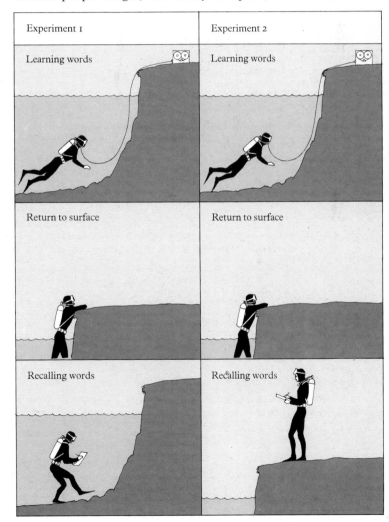

Experiment 1	Experiment 2
Learning words	Learning words
Return to surface	Return to surface
Recalling words	Recalling words

memory store itself. Baddeley argues that the move from one environment to another cannot have erased the memory trace; learning certainly took place, and therefore this form of forgetting can be attributed to some failure in the mechanism of recall. As we shall see later, however, the same may not necessarily be true in cases where brain injury has led to a memory defect.

MEMORY AS A FILING SYSTEM

Alan Baddeley also proposes an interesting parallel between human memory and a library:

> The analogy of the library is actually quite a useful one for conceptualizing human memory. Rather like a library, it's basically a system for storing and subsequently retrieving information. Again like a library it's very important, if you're going to be able to gain access to its information, to be able to store it in an organized and systematic way, and one of the most important characteristics of human memory is that it's organized, that it's meaningful and it's structured. The process of forgetting, if you like, is analogous either to losing the books or losing track of the books and there is a fundamental and long controversy within psychology as to whether forgetting occurs because memory traces fade away or whether in fact they simply become inaccessible. The books are still in the library but they can't be found. The process of retrieval, remembering, getting hold of the information when you want it is analogous to the process whereby a librarian will tell you where to find out information on, for instance, the medical services in the Spanish Civil War. Incidentally, although what the librarian gives you will be a series of books, what he is really providing is an area of knowledge, and the categorization system is concerned with categorizing knowledge, although the books are the way that knowledge is conveyed.

Let us move on. We have looked at learning, and considered the storage of memories, from the point of view of the psychologists. We now look at the work of a neuro-biologist, who tackles the questions with the traditional flair of the experimentalist.

MEMORY PROBLEMS IN THE SEA SLUG

One of the traditional methods of scientific investigation has always been to simplify a problem as far as possible. While it would be absurd to equate Ebbinghaus's learning of simple and nonsensical syllables with the richness of the sort of human memory which would be exemplified by a catalogue of, say, Stanley Holloway's recollections, Ebbinghaus's model was certainly a practical, simple starting place.

The same principle applies in the biological examination of memory. While the human brain contains, according to most estimates, something like 10^{11} or 10^{12} (a million million) brain cells (that is to say approximately the same number as there are stars in our galaxy), yet it is possible to gain some idea of the functioning of the brain by examining animals with far simpler nervous systems.

The flat-worm, the snail and the leech have been popular candidates among neuro-biologists for this reason. A celebrated paper entitled 'Problem Solving in the Leech' attracted unfavourable comment in the United States during one of the US Senate's periodic forays against esoteric science. How equally offensive, then, might appear to be a paper entitled 'Memory Problems in the Sea Slug'? This is an imaginary title, and the animal in question is not strictly speaking a sea slug but what is called a sea hare. Its proper name is *Aplysia*. The nervous system of aplysia, including what might be called its brain or brains, consists of no more than about 10,000 cells, a number which can be viewed without an undue sinking feeling by neuro-biologists.

Eric Kandel, who is Professor of Psychiatry at Columbia University Medical School in New York, takes a very positive stance about his choice of aplysia as a simple, or reductionist, model for comparative investigations aimed at improving our knowledge of human learning.

> It is a very simple animal, and there is no question that human beings have certain memory capabilities that aplysia lacks . . . often that is looked upon as a major weakness in any reductionist approach to the study of memory. But I never thought that that was the critical issue at hand. The question is not whether aplysia can do what humans can do. The question is whether there is anything that humans can do that aplysia can also accomplish, whether there are any aspects of learning that you find to be universally represented in the animal kingdom which both simple and complex animals are capable of carrying out. There's no question about the answer to that.

WHAT IS APLYSIA?

In life aplysia is not an overwhelmingly beautiful animal. It looks like a slug, and is a mottled brownish-purple, about eighteen inches long and can weigh several pounds. It moves, to coin a phrase, sluggishly, and if given what might be termed a noxious stimulus (usually a prod with an electric probe) will emit handsome, purple-coloured ink. In contrast to the animal's appearance in life, aplysia's nervous system dissected out after death is a beautiful thing. The long silver-grey strands of nerve connecting the glowing orange coloured ganglia suggest a biological micro-circuit, so much so that one experimenter refers to his map of the aplysia's nervous system as the wiring diagram.

In experimental terms aplysia has one huge advantage. Its nerve cells are few in number, but enormous in size. Whereas most mammalian brain cells are difficult to see even under a microscope, some of aplysia's cells are so large that they can be seen with the naked eye. Aplysia does not have a brain as such. It has instead a collection of what might be called sub-brains, or ganglia, which control various functions of the animal. A single ganglion controls functions concerned with abdominal parts – rather like a primitive brain. Humans and other animals also have ganglia, but they have the enormous head ganglion we call the brain, which aplysia lacks. Most of what we know about nerve transmission has been studied in the giant nerve fibres of the squid, so for traditional reasons as well as for convenience it seems reasonable for Kandel to use this rather rudimentary nervous system as a model of learning and memory in humans.

Kandel's enthusiasm for aplysia as an experimental subject increased with experience:

> It turned out that aplysia is capable of much richer behaviour and much more elaborate forms of learning than I had initially anticipated. I went to aplysia not because its behavioural repertoire was so rich . . . but because its nervous system was so remarkably attractive, and I thought the limiting factor in the study of behaviour had traditionally been the intractability of the nervous system, not the fact that simple animals don't have behaviour. So I was willing to settle for the relatively modest behaviour that I thought aplysia had in order to take advantage of the enormous power that accrued from having cells that were so large. It turns out that as my colleagues and I have continued to explore aplysia we have found that even simple animals show fairly rich behaviour once you know how to ask the right questions.

The basic technique employed by Kandel is to abstract sets of nerve cells and to study them *in vitro* – that is to say in a glass dish. Electrodes stimulate the cells with a mild electrical current representing nerve signals from sensory nerve cells. The living cells in the dish thus have the same 'behaviour' as they would in the living animal, and are able to respond with signals. These signals, of course, have no end point – they cannot operate muscles because there are no muscles attached; but this is accepted throughout neuro-biology as a model of the events taking place in the living animal.

Kandel and his colleagues have constructed wiring diagrams of parts of the nervous system, showing the nerve cells involved in various behaviours. Some of aplysia's nerve cells – in the abdominal ganglion, for example – are visible to the naked eye, being a little smaller than the head of a pin.

HABITUATION AND SENSITIZATION

The behaviour which has been widely used by Kandel and his colleagues is the so-called 'gill withdrawal reflex'. When an outside part of the animal, the gill, is touched with a glass rod the animal withdraws it. If the prodding is repeated a number of times, the reflex becomes less pronounced – the animal hardly bothers to withdraw its gill, presumably having learnt that the stimulus will do it no harm. Eventually there is almost no reaction to the prodding with the glass rod, and the animal is said to have been habituated. The nervous system has stopped responding to that stimulus.

The cells in their glass dish could be stimulated in the same way, or at least in the same time sequence, as the complete animal,

APLYSIA
One nerve cluster (inset in circle) controls the abdominal muscles. The shaded cell, no R2, is involved in the withdrawal of the gill when it is stimulated.

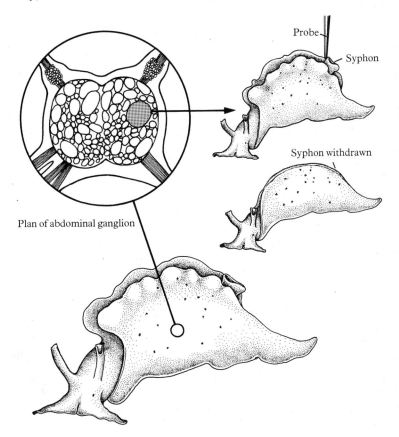

Probe

Syphon

Syphon withdrawn

Plan of abdominal ganglion

and by recording the electric signals given off it was possible to see that repeated stimulation would abolish the reaction of the motor cells which withdraw the gill. After a single training session, giving ten to fifteen stimuli to the living animal, the implanted memory of the stimulus is rather short-lived, lasting only an hour or two. But repeated training sessions cause the habituation to last for weeks. This, believes Kandel, is possibly analogous to short-term and long-term memory in humans.

The opposite form of learning is sensitization. This is demonstrated in aplysia by touching the gill to elicit the gill withdrawal reflex, while at the same time administering a mild electric shock to the animal. This time the animal will learn to withdraw the gill much faster and again the action will be 'remembered' for a period of hours, at least.

Both habituation and sensitization – learning to ignore a stimulus or learning to react very fast to a stimulus – can be brought down to the level of a single synapse. (The *synapse* is the site or point of contact at which one cell communicates with another.) The signal travelling along a nerve is electrical in nature, but when it reaches the synapse it is transformed into a chemical signal which in turn triggers an electrical reaction in the second cell. In habituation, clearly, communication between the two cells at the synapse has been made weaker; in sensitization, communication between the two cells has been made stronger.

At present the chemical processes underlying sensitization are clearer. Kandel and his associates have established to their satisfaction that a larger amount of the 'message chemical' or neuro-transmitter has been released by the first cell across the synapse to the second cell; an amplification, as it were, of the nerve signal from one cell to the next.

PARALLELS IN HUMAN MEMORY

It turns out also that both habituation and sensitization can be produced across the same synapse (not at the same time, of course). If, as appears to be the case, long-term and short-term learning can also use the same synapse, this suggests the possibility that, at least in its early stages, learning in humans for both long-term and short-term memory takes place in the same brain areas – though doubtless across many thousands or millions of times more synapses. The theoretical implications of these discoveries for human memory might be, in a sense, devastating. All the complexities of human memory may, in the last analysis, be reduced to the operation of chemicals at junctions between nerve cells. So, despite our possible feelings to the contrary, there is nothing mystical about a person's sudden flood of recollection, at least in physical (or operational) terms. The complexity of memory, though, will be matched by the complex interchange of signals between our brain cells.

THE ROLE OF NEURO-BIOLOGY

Eric Kandel has high hopes for his approach to the problems of learning and memory.

'If you look at a nerve cell in a snail or in the leech or in a cat, a monkey or human, their signalling properties are extraordinarily similar. The kind of chemicals they use as transmitter substances are very similar, and patterns of synaptic interactions are very similar. Now clearly there will be new mechanisms that one will encounter perhaps only in the human brain. But at the moment our understanding is so primitive that we are grateful for any insight we can have, even insights into the most elementary mental processes. Although at the moment one can't be certain . . . one has reason from just the tradition of biology to feel that the basic processes like these are very likely to be similar in simple animals and in complex ones.' The human brain is the most complex of all brains. If we are to learn about its biological functioning, we must take approaches like Kandel's. There is no other way; but the evolutionary ladder from aplysia to man is immense.

LOSS OF MEMORY

We have seen how our memories can vary in terms of vintage, character and durability. And we have pointed to the sequence of events – selection, storage and recall – that governs our laying down memories. We know, too, that we are capable of forgetting. There are, however, many kinds of forgetting. Most common, perhaps, is the forgetfulness that comes with old age, and many of us have relatives who cannot remember where they left their glasses. (Some of us have much younger relatives who cannot remember where they leave almost all their belongings.) But the degeneration of the brain that occurs as we grow older is not one that is susceptible of measurement while the brain's owner is still living. If it were possible, therefore, to relate the condition of loss of memory to a corresponding, specific deterioration of the brain, we might be able to extend our knowledge of the memory mechanism. The following accounts of two such cases do just that.

AMNESIA – CASE 1: HM

The study of the biology of human memory might almost be said to have begun with an American patient known only by his initials, HM, back in the 1950s. HM was an epileptic, and brain surgeons operated on him in an attempt to relieve that epilepsy.

In the course of the operation the surgeons removed parts of the temporal lobes – among other things HM lost his hippocampus and amygdala, two small parts of the limbic system – and in so doing it seemed that they had deprived HM of the ability to record new memories. He has reasonably good recall of his life up to the time of the operation, and has short-term memory capability, but he has almost no long-term memories following the operation. The psychologists who examined H M concluded, not surprisingly, that these parts are responsible for a great deal of the process of memory in human beings.

H M has the unfortunate distinction of being the most famous amnesic in medical history, and his case is particularly valuable because we know what parts of the brain were removed. Needless to say, the results of the case, once fully appreciated, put an end to such operations. The ill-fated operation did, however, serve to provide physical evidence of the site of some part of the brain's memory apparatus. H M, who was born in 1926, is still alive and well.

AMNESIA – CASE 2: GEORGE

There is on record another case which can be quite precisely described in terms of the wound that caused a memory loss. A psychologist in Southern California, Larry Squire, has a patient (we'll call him George) with a rather specific loss of memory and a fairly precise area of damage.

AMNESIA BY ACCIDENT

There are still puzzling features about George's amnesia, and he is not so clear a case as H M, largely because his injury was not surgical but accidental. The accident happened when George was on Army Service in 1960 in the Azores. George's barrack room mate indulged in horseplay with a small fencing foil, with unfortunate consequences for George:

> I came right round into his lunge . . . I took it right into the left nostril and it went up and punctured my brain. Now, I don't know if it was an inch or an inch and a half or what. I've been told several different stories but we'll leave it go at about an inch . . . I tried getting the foil out of my nose and I couldn't budge it. It was solid. And I said 'Now, look here, Bill, I don't have any pain, I just felt a shock when you hit me, a shock to the brain.' I've never experienced a shock like that before but I told him I felt it. 'And I want you to pull this out for me,' I said, 'I still have feeling but I can't budge this thing.' And he said 'Are you sure?' a couple of times. And I says, 'Yes, I'm positive because now I might feel it in a few minutes and I might pass out. . . .' I said, 'Put your right hand on my forehead holding my head constant and then pull with your left hand, then maybe you can withdraw it.' . . . So he tried it that way and it came right on out, no sweat. I felt nothing but the shock as when it entered, the

same shock when he withdrew it. And I stood there holding my head, trying to shake it around, feel some pain. Now, I had absolutely no reason for feeling it. I didn't feel anything of it, but after a few seconds I felt this warm fluid running up my sleeve and I thought it was going to be blood when I first felt it. I looked at it – a thick clear substance. It seemed it didn't want to stop.

GEORGE AND HIS SECOND SELF

After the accident George did collapse, and he spent months in hospitals. His account of that time is a strange one. He describes feeling that he was sitting in a cinema watching the events that were happening to him apparently happening to someone else on the screen. Sometimes he felt that he was that person, or might be that person, but was never sure. 'At the time of the accident happening I really became somebody outside of my body. I didn't really have control of this character. He walked down the stairwell. He did everything from then on. I didn't really care too much about it because I didn't think it was me.'

About twelve months after the accident George, by now living with his mother in California in a caravan, suddenly connected his two selves and became one person again. He had not made anything like a complete recovery, however, because he could not remember many of the things that he should have remembered. He had become a rather classic case of amnesia following brain damage, and in fact he is crippled by his loss of memory.

WHAT WAS THE DAMAGE?

DAMAGED BRAINS
HM's operation removed the hippocampus and amygdala on both sides (*left*). Compare with George's less extensive damage to the thalamus (*right*).

Since George's injury was accidental it was not easy to be precise about the site and extent of the damage. But the novel technique of Computerized Axial Tomography (CAT) has enabled Larry Squire to identify the area of the injury. In the CAT scan an X-ray camera circles the head and a computer converts its signals into a 'slice' of brain. By comparing such a picture from George's brain with

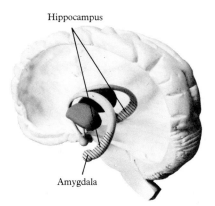

Hippocampus

Amygdala

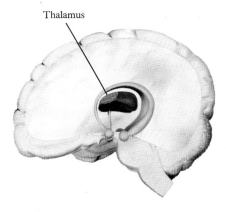

Thalamus

pictures of other brains it was possible to see slight shadows or differences, which were assumed to be the sites of damage. The miniature fencing foil seems to have injured the thalamus, part of the limbic system lying quite close to the hippocampus and amygdala. The injury is on the left-hand side, which will later be seen to be significant in relation to the kind of memory loss that George has.

More exactly, the area damaged was the dorsal medial nucleus of the thalamus.

THE ROLE OF THE THALAMUS

The thalamus is a structure in the mid-brain which seems to be the intersection of a number of different nerve pathways: signals from sight and hearing pass through the thalamus, and it is involved in the control of movement too. But it also receives messages from the limbic system, part of which is the hippocampus, the structure that was removed in HM's case.

So the thalamus is a great junction for many signals and no doubt it also integrates and re-interprets the signals before passing them on to other parts of the brain. Even before George's accident it was known that the thalamus played some part in the memory process. By examining the defects of memory that his injury produced it may be possible to interpret its function.

GEORGE'S MEMORY PROBLEM

Larry Squire found that the differences, clearly shown in psychological tests, between George's recollection of events *after* the accident have something very important to tell us about the way George's injury has affected the memory process.

According to Squire:

> . . . his memory for the times prior to 1960 appears to be perfectly normal, whereas his memory since 1960 is impaired. So this by itself tells us a whole group of facts about the way memory is organized. For example, it tells us that his memory problem, and other amnesics' memory problems, are probably not a deficit in retrieving memory that's there normally; because if it were a deficit in retrieval we'd expect it to apply to all past memories and not just a portion of the past.
>
> So we think . . . that these amnesias constitute a difficulty in laying down new memories and that these brain structures, like the thalamus, are part of the system that's necessary to lay down, or to establish, or to form memories and to elaborate them over a period of time; and that they are not responsible for retrieving

memories or for storing memories . . . we know that the structures that are damaged are not the structures that store memory. These are the structures that are involved in getting a memory system established and the memory system that stores memory is probably functioning, as far as we know, in the cortex, the larger overlying areas of the brain. And that's a very complicated business.

BACK TO BASICS

The distinction between learning, storage and recall to which Larry Squire draws our attention is one that is argued closely among psychologists. Squire's opinion, that it is the learning process rather than the retrieval process which is disrupted in many cases of amnesia, is still a controversial one. Other scientists believe that storage itself has been destroyed. Squire himself makes the point that in order to retrieve there must be a store, and that the circumstances of recall must be affected by the circumstances of learning. It would appear, therefore, that the three phases are interconnected.

TESTING HIS MEMORY

Is it possible to be more precise about the nature of George's memory deficit? We already know that his memory is much worse since the accident and that his memory for events before 1960 is relatively unimpaired. But there are other significant features of his memory deficit which are related to the position of the injury. Remember that the foil damaged part of the *left-hand side* of George's brain, where the centres most concerned with speech and language are to be found.

In the case of George's amnesia, Larry Squire has exhaustively tested his capacity for recollection of verbal versus visual material. The injury in the left side of the brain was likely to make the damage to his verbal processing more acute than the damage to his visual processing. This showed up well in a pair of tests.

In the first test Dr Squire showed George a series of cards with black and white line drawings on them. They were of familiar objects: a bar stool, a coat, a fork, a pie with a piece missing, a boat, a pair of rain boots, a tap and a coat. When questioned about the cards thirty minutes later George could remember seeing them, but had not clearly remembered the object of the test. He thought he had to pick out which pictures he had seen before. The only subject he remembered was the fork. 'Of course, it wasn't what I'd seen before but one was a picture of a fork. I can't recall anything else. Of course at the time I started this I didn't remember a picture of a fork. It just finally came to me.'

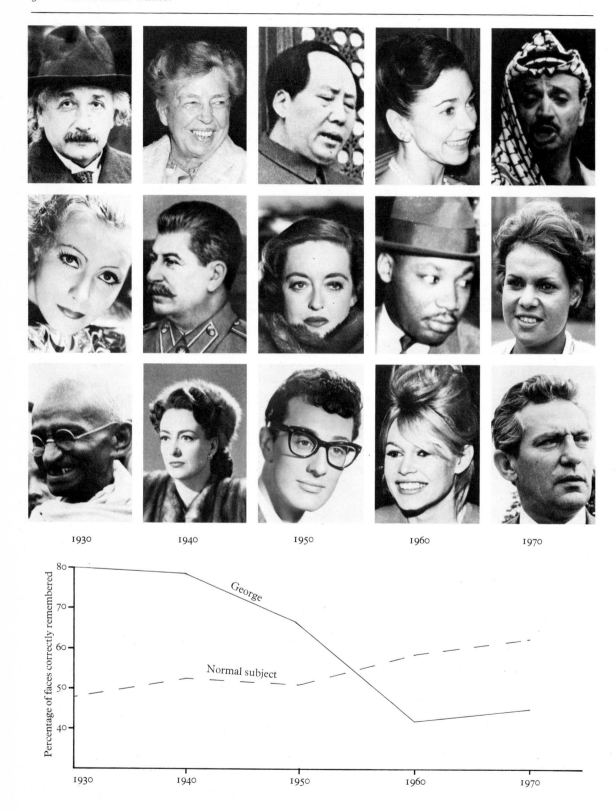

1930   1940   1950   1960   1970

FAMOUS FACES
On a test like this, George's memory is notably better before his accident in 1960 (graph). The reader is invited to test his or her own memory.

So George was at least able to remember one of the objects and was able to remember that he'd seen a set of pictures, even if he wasn't clear why he was being asked to look at them. His visual memory, if not impressive, at least existed.

Next Dr Squire showed him a set of cards with words printed on them. George was required to read out the words: hockey, cradle, badge, magnet, shawl, pepper, soda, throat. After another interval, again half an hour, he was asked (by implication) whether he remembered *either* of the tests:

DR SQUIRE: About an hour ago I think it was we sat here and we talked about some things. I wonder if you could recall what it was we did?

GEORGE: You gave me a bunch of cards to remember different drawings on.

DR SQUIRE: Oh yes.

GEORGE: One was, I think, a couch and I know that isn't what I remembered a few minutes ago but I can't seem to remember what I remembered a few minutes ago. You know, I think it's real strange. I can remember that time of having remembered the other object but I can't remember what the object was now.

DR SQUIRE: Yes. Well, besides these drawings was there any other kind of material that I asked you to look at and remember?

GEORGE: I'm sorry but I can't recall right now if there was any.

DR SQUIRE: Anything else today besides those pictures of objects that you looked at and tried to remember?

GEORGE: Honestly I don't have anything there right now. Maybe there was but I don't remember it.

So George does not even remember seeing the word cards, let alone the words that were printed on them. This seems to be additional evidence that his deficit is in verbal remembering.

George is still living in California, and is still looked after by his mother, although he now lives in his own house, one of a number of units designed for old people. Since 1960 he has been unable to hold down a job, and now attends weekly sessions in craft work as occupational therapy. He does not seem unduly disturbed by his disability, but takes a detached view of himself as a psychological case.

TWO SYSTEMS: VERBAL AND VISUAL

Most of us have, in fact, a system for learning verbal material which is separate from the system we have for learning visual material, and in George's case it is the former which has been damaged irreparably. But before we pass on from George's tragedy, let us consider a distinction between his residual memory capability and the results of experiments on the brain of the rat.

Some recent work has suggested that, at least in the rat, the hippocampus (the area damaged in the case of the famous patient HM) is responsible for spatial learning. Rats with a damaged or removed hippocampus find it difficult to learn their way around a maze which they would master with ease if they were undamaged. There may be some corroboration for the theory of the involvement of the hippocampus in spatial memory in the fact that George's hippocampus is, so far as we know, undamaged.

But this is another of the many controversial areas in the study of memory. It may be reminiscent of phrenology to suggest that one area is concerned with spatial memory, but since we already know that the left-hand side of the brain is concerned with language, perhaps the idea is not so far fetched. There is a further important caveat, however: one may not in such relatively complex cases be able to extrapolate adequately from rat behaviour to human behaviour.

What about people who are trained, by personal inclination or cultural heritage, to remember in particular kinds of ways? We now look at examples of different learning systems in operation.

A MEMORY IN TRAINING

In the case of the underwater learning experiment described earlier, it seemed that recollection of the environment could strengthen encoding in the word-learning task. It has been known for at least two thousand years that learning can be strengthened by setting up interaction between different threads of memory. This is a device employed by professional mnemonists, and was used by Greek and Roman orators to help them remember their speeches without the use of notes.

Such a process can represent an interaction between the systems for learning visual and verbal material which enhances the capacity for learning, and usually results in improved learning of verbal material, the mnemonists' stock-in-trade. We came across the technique in action. Today's mnemonists use the old orators' system for their own purposes. We met an amateur mnemonist, Trevor Emmott, who based his system on a code which can be learned, as he says, as easily as morse code.

It's quite an old idea. The version that I adopted dates from the 1840s. It's really just a code which enables you to convert the ten digits into sounds and then you convert those sounds into words. So, for example, the figure one is represented by the sound of the letter T, three is M, four is R, five is L and so on. If I wanted to

THE FIGURE ALPHABET

The code used by Trevor Emmott to form words and help him memorize numbers. Vowels have no numerical value and can be used in any position. The example shows a number coded as letters, then words and pictures combined into a scene.

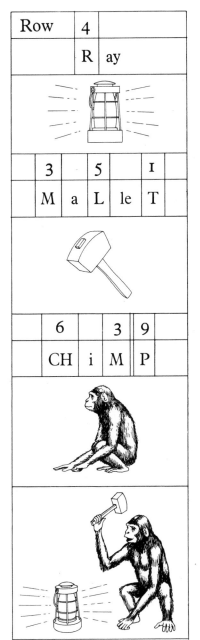

Row	4		
	R	ay	

3	5		I
M	a	L	le	T

6		3	9
CH	i	M	P

remember a simple number, 32, and used this system I would first of all convert that into the sound M and N and then I would add vowels which don't have any numerical value and I would build those sounds up into a word such as MAN or MOON or MINE or OMEN. And then of course I've got a word which I can turn into a picture.

Normally Trevor will ask you to give him a series of digits or numbers, and when he has memorized them, using his sound and picture technique, he will ask you to show him the next number. We gave him a more difficult problem. We took him up to Lytham St Anne's where ERNIE the Premium Bond computer does nothing else but print out strings of random numbers. ERNIE does this at his own speed, which is one set of six numbers every five seconds, a faster speed than was comfortable for Trevor. But he (Trevor that is, not ERNIE) gamely agreed to give it a try.

We asked ERNIE to deliver six sets of six digits each – thirty-six numbers in all. Trevor concentrated hard as he watched ERNIE's teleprinter rattling out the numbers. Then he tried to recollect them. 'Well, I'll try that group of six starting with the first one. That is 859595; 606072; 443414; 351639; 4 – no, I'm having difficulty with the fifth group. Let me just try the sixth and I can come back to the fifth. That I think is 446929. Then, yes, the fifth group, that was 790069.'

Trevor was subsequently able to recall the numbers in any order, back to front or even diagonally by using his mnemonic technique. What was interesting, though, was the row which Trevor failed to remember. Had his system failed, or was the presentation simply too fast?

I think the reason was that I was trying to split the six digits into two groups of three and to get a single word for each three-figure group. Now I did that in the fifth row with the first three figures easily. 790 got the word COPIES. I thought about a photocopying machine producing copies. But 069 I found difficult on the spur of the moment. I couldn't get a single word and I spent a little too long trying to get a single word so eventually I had to give up and divide it into two words and I got SASH and PIE. Now there's no great difficulty linking together those three words, COPIES, SASH, PIE, and also linking them to the peg number but I spent a little too long over it. I was rather worried about the passage of time and I didn't form a very strong interaction between the elements. I think that was the problem.

However, the trick worked well enough, and Trevor is now going through his paces for psychologists at Birkbeck College in London.

It would be tempting to think that memory problems could be helped by the use of such techniques – that combinations of the memory systems could aid the overall working of a memory – and in some cases this may be possible. But in George's case, where one memory system seems in any case to be defective, it is probably that the interaction could not be achieved, and that no memory improvement would result.

A Sense of Place

We follow Trevor Emmott's considerable expertise in verbal learning with something completely different. Psychologists have been investigating the extent to which different human cultures may affect the manner in which memories develop, and the roles which the verbal and visual systems play.

Judith Kearins, a psychologist at the University of Western Australia in Perth, has made a particular study of aspects of the memory of the aboriginal people of the Australian outback. It is common knowledge that the aborigine can find his way around the trackless wastes of the Continent with no apparent effort. Yet this astonishing skill is at odds with the poor performance of aboriginal children in routine intelligence tests at school. Judith Kearins wanted to find out more.

'In the past, aboriginal children have always fared badly on cognitive tests and I was interested in trying some task which was from their side of the fence. I saw it as a very interesting problem, really. What would happen if you tried to get aboriginal kids to perform on a task which affected cognitive skills or ways of thinking that they used in their own cultures, rather than tests from within western culture?'

Judith Kearins tested children of various ages. She has worked in truly remote desert regions as well as in sparsely populated regions nearer towns, and she has tested children with an almost entirely traditional upbringing as well as children whose upbringing on the outskirts of urban areas has been similar to white children from similar environments. As far as possible, she has paired her groups of aboriginal children with similar groups of white children in order to draw reliable scientific conclusions from her tests. Although her interest is spatial memory, and she believes it to be relevant to finding one's way in the desert, she points out that all she is testing is the ability of children to do her tests.

Judith Kearins is very conscious that she is an outsider in these circumstances, and she has taken great care to integrate herself into the society of the aboriginal children, to be seen by all the people who want to satisfy their curiosity, and to answer all the children's questions about herself. Then she can set to work.

The tests that Judy Kearins uses are not difficult to understand. They are based on a sort of 'Kim's Game' involving four small trays, each divided into from twelve to twenty compartments. Each tray contains a different set of objects. The first has small man-made objects, like an eraser, a thimble, a ring, a pair of scissors and so on, which are likely to be familiar to white children. The second has about twenty natural objects likely to be familiar to desert children – a feather, a rock, a leaf, a small skull and so on. The third has twelve small rocks simply varying in size, shape and colour. The fourth is a set of small bottles, man-made, of course, and all similar; they are familiar to white children, but hard to describe. Judy shows each tray in turn to the child she is testing. Then, asking the child to cover up his or her eyes, she jumbles the objects and asks her subject to replace the objects in their original positions. In her tests she always found that the achievement of the aboriginal children was greater than the achievement of matched white children.

> I've tested children between the ages of about six and sixteen years and they always perform better than white Australian children. . . . They perform about three years ahead of the white Australian children, so that an aboriginal child of about seven years would perform as well as a ten-year-old white Australian child. Not quite as well, but it's about a three-year difference. This is a highly significant difference and it exists on all of my spatial memory tasks between the two groups and at all ages, so in that sense it's real, it's trustworthy. . . .

One of the other differences that Judy Kearins found was that while white Australian children mutter to themselves while they try to do the tests, the aboriginal children remain quite silent and impassive. This leads her to believe that the white Australian children are using what she calls a naming strategy, whereas the aboriginal children are using a purely visual strategy to accomplish the task.

> Aboriginal children have been said, along with other hunters and gatherers, to be brought up with independence for a long time, and I'm sure it's the case with aboriginal people today, even in the non-traditional setting. And this implies quite a lot of interesting things for the way they learn to think. . . . They are not talked at to the same extent that white children are. They're not expected to obey verbal commands and therefore they are free to use visual processing, watching strategies, for all of their early years. And from what I've seen they really use vision a great deal in ordinary everyday interchanges. They aren't expected to speak if they don't feel like it, and they certainly aren't expected to listen. The fact that we are means that we grow up using linear

processing in verbal habits which aboriginal children probably encounter for the first time in school.

Judy Kearins's test results tend to confirm the established existence of the separate memory systems for visual and verbal reasoning, and at the same time indicate that our cultural upbringing not only affects the way we think but also the way we remember things. This leads us on, in the closing sections of this chapter, to a survey of the latest developments in memory research.

MEMORY, AND THE CHEMISTRY OF THE BRAIN

It is in brain chemistry that the greatest strides have been taken in the last few years. In the early 1970s there were some attempts to reduce the idea of learning to an almost absurdly simplistic level. It was suggested that chemical changes of some sort, in protein or in the nucleic acid, stored the memory trace. Claims were made that learning for mazes, for example, could be transferred from one animal by feeding or injecting a second animal with chemicals extracted from the former's brain. The experiments proved difficult to replicate, and today there is probably no scientist who retains quite those views. That brain chemicals are involved is not, of course, in doubt, but it is their action in passing messages at the synapse that currently absorbs most effort.

Perhaps the current concentration on biochemistry has tended to reduce the amount of work done on the location of the memory trace. This is still thought likely to be stored in the cerebral cortex – possibly in dispersed form. The Canadian neurologist, Wilder Penfield, during brain operations was able to elicit what appeared to be memories by stimulating the exposed cortex of his patient's brain. Some amazing apparent recalls took place, but these experiments have been difficult to reproduce, and today there is some doubt as to the nature of the 'recall' which Penfield's patients exhibited. Certainly it is possible to localize some functions in different parts of the brain, but the localization of memory is much more in question.

CHEMISTRY, ANATOMY, AND A NEW THEORY

Recently a new hypothesis seems to link chemical and anatomical studies. It comes from the University of Irvine in California and the leader of the team concerned is Gary Lynch.

Lynch has been looking at the hippocampus of the rat. A new technique involves taking slices of a hippocampus rapidly separated from the brain of a freshly killed rat. (The nerve cells in the hippocampus are very regularly arranged and therefore one slice is very like another.) A slice can be kept alive in a nutrient solution and, by the use of electrodes, the slice of tissue can be stimulated to

THE MEMORY GAME
Judy Kearins uses displays like these for children to memorize. The all-different set is easy to name in words, but the all-similar set of rocks is difficult.

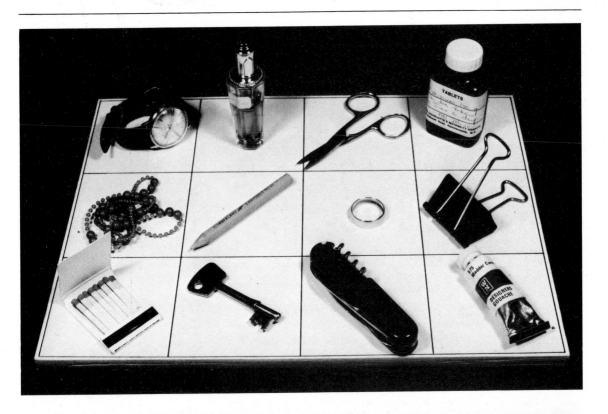

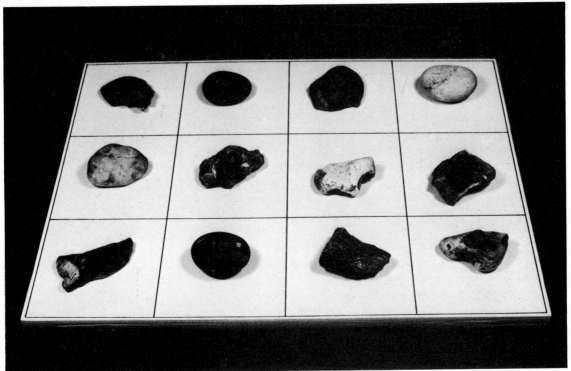

respond with nerve signals. While Kandel was stimulating preparations containing only a few cells of aplysia, Lynch is stimulating preparations containing millions of cells. Like Kandel, he finds that messages – the output signals – pass more easily after repetitive stimulation of cells, and sees this as a simple model of learning. The term he uses, though, is 'long-term potentiation'.

Lynch's technique is immensely laborious. He stimulates the slice of hippocampus with a very mild electric shock until he believes that synaptic changes have occurred, on the evidence of his monitoring equipment. As soon as this has been achieved the hippocampus slice is frozen and photographed under the electron microscope. Serial pictures are taken right through the slice, and examined to see if the synapses show any sign of change. And Lynch and his colleagues believe that they have seen such changes that are significant.

CHANGING SYNAPSES
Shaft synapses which Gary Lynch believes show an increase in number after electrical stimulation. The first picture has been modified to show a possible 'before' state. It is impossible to take pictures of the same slice before and after stimulation, because the process used to make electron microscope pictures destroys the slice. The real experiment is based on statistical methods, comparing stimulated with unstimulated cells.

Let me first say that the connections between nerve cells in the hippocampus are of two groups. The first is what we call a spine contact. Now by that we mean that the input, that is to say the axon from one cell connects with a target cell via a protuberance on the target cell. This business is called a spine. Ninety-seven per cent of the contacts in the hippocampal formation are of the spine variety and the great mass of contacts between nerve cells in your cerebral cortex are of the spine variety. We find that, following this repetitive stimulation that leads to the long-term potentiation, these spines have changed their shape.

Now, let me emphasize that that's a deduction from the data. We know that the spine is changed and from careful analysis . . . of that data we believe that the nature of that change is that the thing becomes rounder. There are bio-physical reasons as to why a rounder spine would be a more efficient spine.

We've also found a second kind of structural change that is more exotic, and I would say in all frankness more difficult to swallow. There is another category of dendrite (*the receptor fibre of the nerve cell*) in the hippocampus. There is no spine in this type. The contact is made directly on to the dendrite. About three per cent of the contacts are of this variety and we believe that this three per cent is on a specialized type of cell. And after the repetitive stimulation and the long-term potentiation we find that there is a thirty to forty per cent increase in this category of contact.

Now, we have struggled with alternative explanations for this phenomenon. We've sought to find other interpretations of our data and I really can't come up

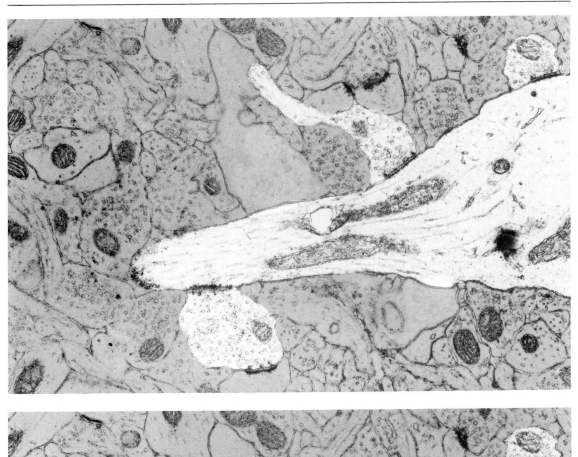

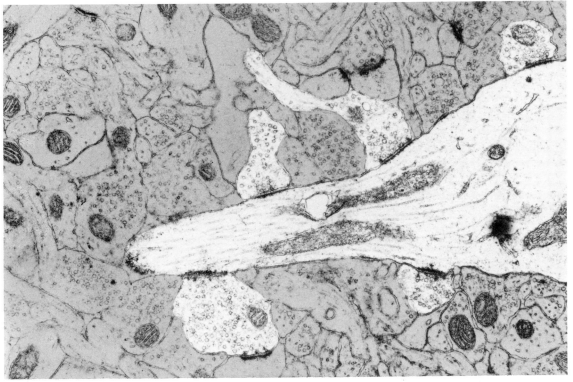

with anything other than the idea that the repetitive stimulation is causing an increase in the frequency of this kind of contact, which is to say that the repetitive stimulation is producing new synapses. The data here is very compelling. If our interpretation of that data is correct it is saying that half a second of activity on this input is causing the creation quite literally of new connections in the brain, and I imagine that this is perhaps the most extraordinary result to come out of our work. Now, I hasten to add that we knew in advance that the hippocampus had the capacity to build new connections, as does the cerebral cortex. But to produce the phenomenon with half a second of stimulation and to have it appear within ten minutes is rather remarkable.

A MEMORY DRUG?

After discovering these structural changes, which continue to confound a number of other scientists, Lynch and his colleagues went on to try to find out why they took place. They believe the changes are linked with an enzyme which seems to affect the ability of the synapses to receive chemical messages from other cells. Says Lynch:

> We are searching for a biochemical machine that is responsible for these alterations in structure, and we have found some drugs that, at least in the test tube, begin to manipulate that machine. If indeed the changes that we are seeing here are changes that the animal actually uses in the biological and psychological universe, and they are caused by the effects or the underlying mechanisms that we suspect they're caused by, then I think there's a possibility that there'll be a pharmacology directed at this sort of thing and I can't predict the significance of that. Potentially I think it could be staggering. The brain is losing millions of neurons from the time it is eighteen years old. Probably the brain adjusts to this by making these kinds of structural changes. Now if we can find ways to influence the process, to facilitate it, then I think the clinical edge would be tremendous; but at this point of course that's science fiction.

FOOD FOR THOUGHT

So memory, at least in lower animals and possibly therefore in humans as well, can be reduced to the happenings at a synapse or at least at a thousand or a million synapses. And these happenings may be influenced by the sort of drug that Lynch talks about. All the data we have from these and hundreds of similar experiments is indirect. It may not apply to human beings, or at least, there is no direct evidence to say that it does. The only evidence we have of a direct link between memory and the brain comes from cases such as those of HM and George. And the human brain is so infinitely more complex than the brain of any other animal that the lessons we learn from aplysia or from rats are difficult to apply to human beings.

The human mind, whatever we may mean by that term, is infinitely resourceful, and one of its resources is introspection. The innumerable galaxy of nerve cells that George has in his skull somehow permits him to find some degree of consolation for even such a dreadful injury as his.

'There are, I guess, many missing pieces but I don't remember that I miss them. I don't remember what it is I'm missing, so I don't pay too much attention to it. The only reason I say that is because there is a lot more to life than what I have been saying, and I'm saying everything that I can remember. So that means there is a heck of a lot more that I am not saying.'

Like a man whose leg has been amputated, George can make the best of his situation. He, too, has lost a part of his body, but when those cells were killed, part of his individual memories died too. George's memories, like yours and ours, are contained in the amazing tissue of the brain. That it is so, increases our sense of wonder at the capacity of nature to enclose so much into our small skulls.

Forward from Memory

Even memory cannot function in isolation as the dictator of the brain's activities. All our capacities may depend on it, but it depends on them, too. We shall see that we need memory to speak, to see, to move and to feel emotions; but these faculties feed back into memory: without vision we cannot remember sights, and without language we cannot remember words. The functions of the brain can be listed separately, but it is only when they are integrated together that a brain becomes human. We will see in Chapter 7 that the dominant left half of the brain contains language. Since it is in language that we express our thoughts and explain the world to ourselves and others, we can see it as a central pivot of our humanity. It is to the understanding of language that we turn next.

CHAPTER 2

LANGUAGE

Language is used for many of the more precise and dry aspects of human expression: the law, scientific exposition, logic. It is therefore tempting to see it as a precise device for communication. This chapter illustrates the strange balance that exists in the brain between this precision, which determines the unyielding grammar of language, and the human tendency to use words and sentences to mean whatever we want them to mean.

WORDS AND LANGUAGE

The words you are reading now have already become nerve signals. They are tracing fixed pathways in your brains which, if damaged, would render even the best prose meaningless. Yet they are also tracing other pathways and calling up other associations which are unique to you, your brain and its memories, intentions and desires. And therefore each individual's interpretation of language is unique and personal.

Other animals have the capacity to fear, to move, to learn, perhaps to love, even to use tools. Only man speaks a language. The study of language is for some philosophers the basis of their theories. Language is seen by them as a model for thought, not just its vehicle. But when we see it in relationship to the brain, language may not be quite as we imagine it.

When he wrote *Through the Looking Glass* Lewis Carroll was playing with the idea of language representing the real world, the paradox of its apparent precision existing alongside a capacity for allusion. Perhaps this was because Charles Lutwidge Dodgson, the academic, rather than Lewis Carroll, the writer, was a mathematician: and mathematics is a peculiarly precise language. Alice's conversation with Humpty Dumpty is a set of variations on the theme of words and their meaning.

> HUMPTY DUMPTY: . . . There's glory for you!
> ALICE: I don't know what you mean by 'glory'.
> HUMPTY DUMPTY: Of course you don't – till I tell you.
> I meant 'there's a nice knock-down argument'.

ALICE: But 'glory' doesn't mean 'a nice knock-down argument'.

HUMPTY DUMPTY: When *I* use a word, it means just what I choose it to mean – neither more nor less.

ALICE: The question is, whether you *can* make words mean so many different things.

HUMPTY DUMPTY: The question is, which is to be the master – that's all. . . . They've a temper, some of them – particularly verbs: they're the proudest – adjectives you can do anything with, but not verbs – however, *I* can manage the whole lot of them! Impenetrability! That's what I say!

ALICE: Would you tell me, please, what that means?

HUMPTY DUMPTY: Now you talk like a reasonable child. . . . I meant by 'impenetrability' that we've had enough of that subject, and it would be just as well if you'd mention what you mean to do next, as I suppose you don't mean to stop here all the rest of your life.

ALICE: That's a great deal to make one word mean.

HUMPTY DUMPTY: When I make a word do a lot of work like that . . . I always pay it extra.

✳   ✳   ✳

ALICE: You seem very clever at explaining words, Sir. Would you kindly tell me the meaning of the poem called 'Jabberwocky'?

HUMPTY DUMPTY: Let's hear it. I can explain all the poems that ever were invented – and a good many that haven't been invented just yet.

ALICE: ''Twas brillig, and the slithy toves
Did gyre and gimble in the wabe:
All mimsy were the borogoves,
And the mome raths outgrabe.'

HUMPTY DUMPTY: . . . there are plenty of hard words there. 'Brillig' means four o'clock in the afternoon – the time when you begin *broiling* things for dinner.

ALICE: That'll do very well . . . and what are 'toves'?

HUMPTY DUMPTY: Well, 'toves' are something like badgers – they're something like lizards – and they're something like corkscrews . . . they make their nests under sundials – also they live on cheese. . . .

ALICE: And 'the wabe' is the grass plot round a sundial, I suppose?

HUMPTY DUMPTY: Of course it is. It's called 'wabe', you know, because it goes a long way before it, and a long way behind it –

ALICE: And a long way beyond it on each side.

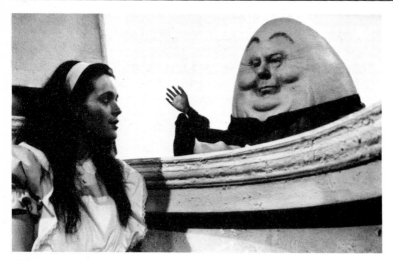

Humpty Dumpty seems, at first reading, to be talking nonsense, but as we examine our own use of language later in the chapter it will be clear that he is a philosopher of some distinction.

Even though many of Humpty Dumpty's words are obviously nonsense words, it is still possible for Alice and for us to identify them as particular parts of speech. So 'slithy' is an adjective, 'gyre' is a verb, and the 'wabe' is a noun. (Notice how cleverly and logically he justifies it: 'way before', 'way behind'.) We know this because of the way the sentence is arranged, and the order of the words. So syntax and grammar, as well as words themselves, contribute to meaning. And, of course, syntax varies from language to language. The order of words in Latin, or German, or French, is different from the order of words in a comparable English sentence. The languages of man are almost infinite in their variability. But the ability to speak and understand them is located in the same parts of the brain, whether the language is a New Guinea dialect or classical Spanish. The ability to use language in its latent complexity is already built into our brain. The study of the brain's language capabilities requires some notion, some model or metaphor to explain how it might be working.

A PRIMITIVE METAPHOR

The gardens of French aristocrats of the seventeenth century were frequently decorated with elaborate fountains. It was not surprising, perhaps, that René Descartes took his metaphor for at least one of the brain's functions from these joyful waterworks. He proposed that the brain operated the muscles on the hydraulic system, springing from the fluid-filled spaces or ventricles within the brain, with tiny hydraulic tubes (nerves) running down to the muscles, rather like the hydraulic brake lines in a modern car. He suggested that the fluid operated the muscles just as a head of water operates a hydraulic machine. Given the time of its origin, the theory was not so unsophisticated. Indeed, large nerves do seem to be tube-like. But Descartes' hydraulic brain was discarded when, a century later, Galvani discovered that nerves seemed to use electricity for transmitting their information from brain to muscles. When, a hundred years later still, Bell invented the telephone, the analogy of the brain as a machine seemed even better. And a machine that converted speech into electricity and back again was surely a superb analogy for the brain, and even suggested its control of language. So the brain, thought scientists, became a sort of exchange, somehow the interface between the input of hearing and the output of speech. The analogy, of course, broke down because it still needed a human agency to react to the input: all a telephone line does is carry signals. When another hundred years had passed, a computer could be employed to do that job at least in theory; now computers are just beginning to process language like humans. But the telephone analogy does indeed have an overwhelming clarity. And it does turn out that breaking connections in the brain will interfere with the brain's processing of language and speech.

CONNECTIONS AND DISCONNECTIONS

If the local telephone exchange were to break down, due to a disconnection in one of the lines, and if the engineers were also on strike, it might be necessary for an unskilled artificer to attempt to mend the wire and restore the function of the telephone system. In the process of doing so, he would necessarily have to discover how the telephone wires were connected one to another, and see something of the pattern of the whole system. That is the aim of the modern neurologist when he examines a patient whose language system has broken down as a result of brain damage. The neurologist cannot, alas, restore the connection in the damaged brain, but by examining very precisely the sort of defect the damage – the break in the connection – has produced, he may gain an inkling of the way in which the brain produces language.

Norman Geschwind, Putnam Professor of Neurology at Harvard University, is one of the world's most distinguished neurologists, and he has made a special study of language. As if to prove this he has a fund of comic anecdotes, and lists his main hobby as argument. Most of his patients are inmates of Boston hospitals, including the Beth Israel Hospital, and it was there that he met one of them, Charles Landry. Somewhere in Mr Landry's brain, the connections have been broken.

Charles Landry was born in New England. He lied about his age, joined the US Marines at 16 and was soon in the Intelligence Corps where he learnt five foreign languages. Back in civilian life, he became one of the most successful criminal lawyers on Cape Cod, with a practice in the small town of Hyannis, not far from the

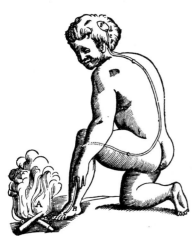

MECHANICAL MAN
In the 17th century René Descartes proposed that heat from a fire was transferred by a change in pressure along tubes which connected up with the spaces or ventricles within the brain. Signals to the muscles were sent down from the brain by a similar mechanism. Although we now know that it is the nerves which transfer all high-speed signals to and fro, the mechanistic approach is still used to explain the brain's comprehension and production of language.

Kennedy estate. In May 1977 Charles Landry had a stroke. He was 45 years old. On admission to hospital, he appeared to the doctor as healthy and relatively alert, and in no acute distress. But he had 'expressive aphasia', meaning he could only speak a word or two, though he followed commands well. He seemed to comprehend, and nodded appropriately. That was the beginning of a hard fight for Charles Landry to recover his speech. Norman Geschwind did not see him until February 1978.

The stroke affected the left side of Charles's brain, and now his whole right side is almost paralysed. (The left side of the brain controls much of the right side of the body, and vice versa.) Otherwise, he seems in fair physical trim. He manages to fire a sporting rifle with the aid of a sling, using his left hand, and he goes sailing with his family. It is his speech which is still most noticeably affected, though like his other disabilities it is a good deal better than it was in 1977. It is very halting and full of pauses, which we will not attempt to reproduce. How did the stroke happen?

> It was the day before hunting started, and I was in Great Barrington, and I took my car keys out with my left hand and I fell to the floor. A strange sort of feeling came over me. The right side of me was paralysed and I couldn't speak. The ambulance driver put my head on one side and I was talking, but nothing was coming out, nothing. I was in shock. Then we got to the hospital and they did not know what to make of it. I don't know what happened to me and then my sons told me that I'm going to another hospital.

AN ANALYTICAL EXAMINATION

When Professor Geschwind examines patients like Charles Landry he uses nothing but a set of questions. With them alone he dissects the brain as efficiently and accurately as a surgeon. He is looking for the 'telephone' connections in Charles's brain and in particular for the places where the connections are broken.

Even if Professor Geschwind knew nothing about the stroke and its location he would still be able to deduce that the brain damage was on the left side. He owes this knowledge to the nineteenth-century pioneers of neurology to whom he is more than willing to pay his debts. In the case of language, the first of these pioneers, Paul Broca, was born in France in 1824. He was both a distinguished surgeon and anthropologist. The son of a country doctor, Broca went to Paris as a medical student, and a poor one at that, in the 1840s. His first post as a doctor was at the Bicêtre Hospital, a lunatic asylum, where his chief, Dr Leuret, had a special interest in the anatomy of the brain. Broca survived the revolution of 1848, and on the return of peace began to devote himself to

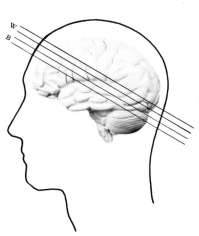

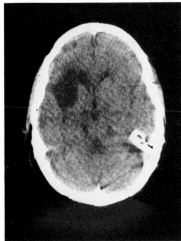

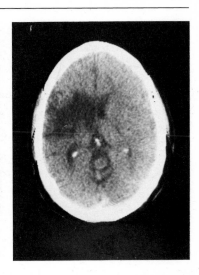

A DAMAGED BRAIN

The dark regions on these computerized X-rays show where Charles Landry's brain 'died' after his stroke. The damaged area is about the size of an egg. The slice on the left is taken from the front (at the top) to the back of his head and passes through Broca's area, one of the major language areas.

On the right, the X-ray slice was taken slightly lower and shows that the other main language area towards the back, Wernicke's area (*see page 51*), is undamaged. Mr Landry's strange language disabilities can be related to the position of his brain damage: in the region of Broca's area, but deeper into the brain.

various studies, including rickets, cancer, hypnotism and anthropology. But his most famous contribution to medical history was the localization of brain function. Earlier in the century, the so-called science of phrenology had suggested that different areas, or bumps, on the head could be associated with various human capabilities, including imagination, love, hate and criminality. This theory was not well received in conventional medical circles, and it must therefore have been with some courage that Broca put forward the theory that language was associated with a particular region of the brain.

BROCA'S AREA

He heard somebody (perhaps interested in phrenology) give a lecture about the shape of the skull and its relationship to the brain. The lecturer said that the frontal part of the brain was involved in language. Broca, being rather sceptical about this, went back to his own ward. He had a patient there with very severe language disturbance as a result of brain damage, and Broca examined him with great care. It happened that the patient died shortly afterwards. When Broca took out the brain, he was rather excited to discover that in fact there was damage in its frontal region. Everyone would have guessed that language was everywhere in the brain. Language is after all something that depends entirely on the environment in which we grow up, so in the first place everyone speaks a different language. But Broca showed in that case and many other cases that damage only to certain regions leads to disturbances of language.

The brain of Broca's patient, who was called Tan because 'tan' was the only word he could say, was preserved in a glass jar and placed in the museum of the Dupuytren Hospital in Paris. For many years it was forgotten and the museum became derelict.

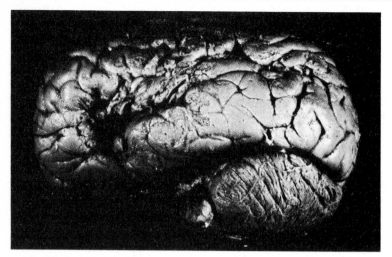

TAN'S BRAIN
This brain, preserved for over 120 years, was the piece of evidence for the localization of language. The damage near the front of the left hemisphere can be clearly seen. Patients with such damage have a very limited vocabulary and lose much of their grammar.

Eventually it even seemed that the brain had disappeared, and with its disappearance all that remained was Broca's 1861 publication, so controversy raged over Broca's theory, even though he had examined many other cases. With the original brain of Tan lost, there were bound to be doubts among those scientists who did not believe, despite Broca's paper, that language could be localized to a particular place in the brain. Then, only a few years ago, the museum curator started systematically to examine the collection of human relics in the mouldering cellars of the museum. They are a gruesome selection of almost every conceivable part of the human anatomy, with almost every conceivable deformity. There, on a dusty shelf right at the back of the cellar was Tan's brain. When its re-discoverer looked at it, the dark area of damage appeared to be in the expected place. Such a precious specimen could not be dissected, and some doubt remained over Broca's findings. Then two Parisian professors, Signoret and Borie, suggested using a new technique: Computerized Axial Tomography, the CAT scan, which shows damage by taking three-dimensional X-ray photographs of the brain without injuring it in any way. When the X-rays were examined, Broca's thesis was vindicated. The damage to Tan's brain was in just the place he had described, towards the front of the left hemisphere. The embalmer, perhaps Broca himself, who had embalmed many a corpse during the bloody revolution of '48, had done his work well and despite the great age of the brain, there was no indication of any other significant damage. Certainly damage to this area would result in gross *speech defects*. But Broca claimed that they were *language defects* and as Professor Geschwind pointed out to us, that would mean that if the patient's speech was transcribed, and all the inaccuracies of particular sounds were taken out, the language would be incorrect either in grammar or in word choice. At that time everybody thought that each language had its own distinctive grammar, but remarkably, it turns out that damage to certain limited regions of the brain produces effects on grammar or word choice everywhere in the world.

The region which Broca discovered in Tan's brain to have been involved in language disturbance is now known as Broca's area, and the disorder of language associated with the damage is known as Broca's aphasia. The patient speaks slowly with enormous effort, and sounds are poorly produced. But he also talks very ungrammatically, leaving out the small words, such as 'if', 'and' or 'but', so that his speech sounds like a telegram. However, the patient usually has the same gaps in his comprehension of language that he hears spoken.

WERNICKE'S AREA

There is a second area on the left side of the brain connected with disorders of language, Wernicke's area. It is further back than Broca's area and is named after Carl Wernicke who published his ideas in 1874, when he was only 26. Wernicke is perhaps Geschwind's hero. This may be because, for the forty years from about 1920 until Geschwind and his teachers re-read them in 1961, the theories of Wernicke and the other proponents of the theory of localization of language function had been severely questioned. They were to prove an inspiration to Geschwind and to his colleagues and successors in this area of neurology.

A patient with damage in Wernicke's area is almost the exact opposite of a Broca's aphasic. His speech will, in extreme cases, be faster than normal. He will talk a great deal, with a normal melody of speech, the sounds will be perfectly all right, and the grammar will be normal. The abnormality is that the patient has enormous difficulty in finding the right word. So he tends to produce a lot of roundabout descriptions. When trying to say, 'flower' he may say, 'Well, you know, the thing that grows out there,' pointing to the

LANGUAGE AREAS
In the 1870s Carl Wernicke, working in Breslaw, associated some of his patients strange jargon speech with a certain region of the brain, also on the left side, but further back than Broca's area. Today we know that such patients have correct grammar, but construct a sort of 'word salad' with many roundabout descriptions, and may even use non-words like 'fleaber' or 'sodent'. Their speech may at first be humorous, but soon frustrates and embarrasses listener and patient alike.

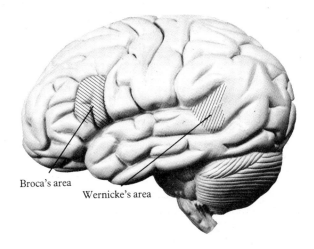

Broca's area

Wernicke's area

garden. He may try to say, 'aeroplane' and say, 'The thing, you know, that goes up in the air,' and he may replace perfectly good English words with other words, such as 'knife' for 'fork'. Sometimes he puts in words which seem to be totally unrelated. One of Professor Geschwind's patients, when shown a coin, said, 'This is an Argentinian rifle.' Norman Geschwind had no idea what the relationship was between that and 'coin'. Sometimes they even produce words that do not exist, like 'fleaber' or 'sodent', saying, for example, 'Well, I was up at the fleaber, and they had a bunch of them there, because the sodent wasn't right. I knew if it wasn't right, well then they had to mark it down.' With language like that one often has no notion at all what the patient is trying to say. However, those who work with them or care for them seem to be able to work a lot of it out, just through experience.

ARCHAEOLOGY OF THE BRAIN Tan's brain on the shelf in the cellars of the Musée Dupuytren in Paris where it was discovered by the curator, Professor R. Abelanet. The tissue was so well preserved after many years that it could be subjected to the most modern investigative techniques, and reveal the damage first seen by Paul Broca in 1861.

THE LEFT HALF

Both major language areas are in the left hemisphere in all but about one person in twenty. Until about ten years ago no one could see any reason for this, then Norman Geschwind and a colleague, Walter Levitsky, decided to examine human brains to see whether the language-dominant left half was in any way discernibly different from the right half. It had long been assumed that, despite the functional differences, no gross difference visible to the naked eye could be seen. But Geschwind and Levitsky's rather straightforward examination, using instruments no more sophisticated than a camera and a ruler, showed quite distinct anatomical differences in the cortex on the left side. In particular, part of Wernicke's area seemed generally to be larger on the left side. It was later discovered that this asymmetry could also be detected in the human foetus, indicating that the enlargement in the left side of the brain cannot entirely be the result of language learning in children but must be partly 'built-in'. The organization of cells in the left half of the brain is different from that in corresponding areas on the right. Even so the right hemisphere can take over language in children under the age of eight who have operations to remove the left hemisphere, if it is severely damaged.

Curiously enough, other mammals also appear to have some degree of brain asymmetry. Since no other species is known to use language, it is hard to ascribe any such asymmetry to the same basic causes as the asymmetry in human brains. But some tasks involving hearing appear to be directed more to the left cerebral cortex in some species of monkey; and in some song birds the left side of the brain is more important for singing. However, it would be rash to assume any straightforward connection between these features of animal brains and the anatomical differences, let alone the functional differences, between the two halves of the human brain.

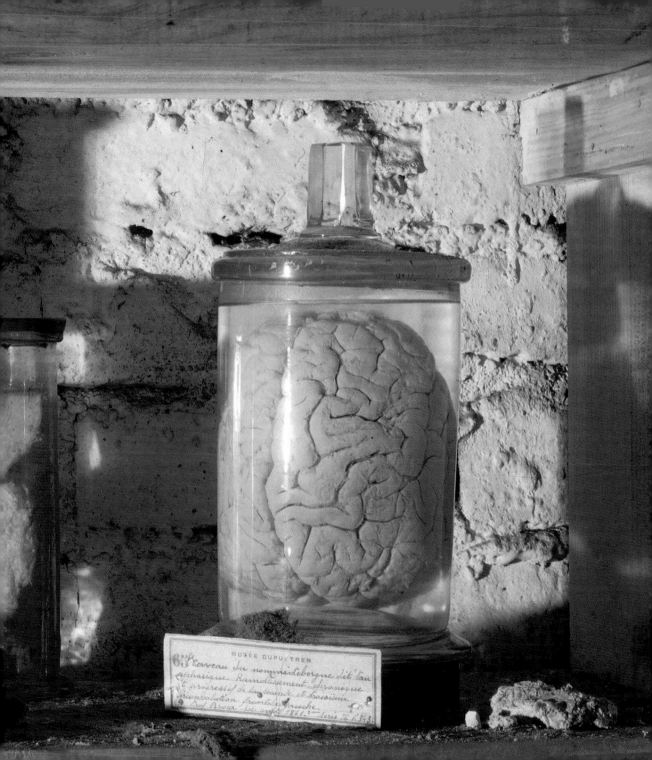

MUSÉE DUPUYTREN

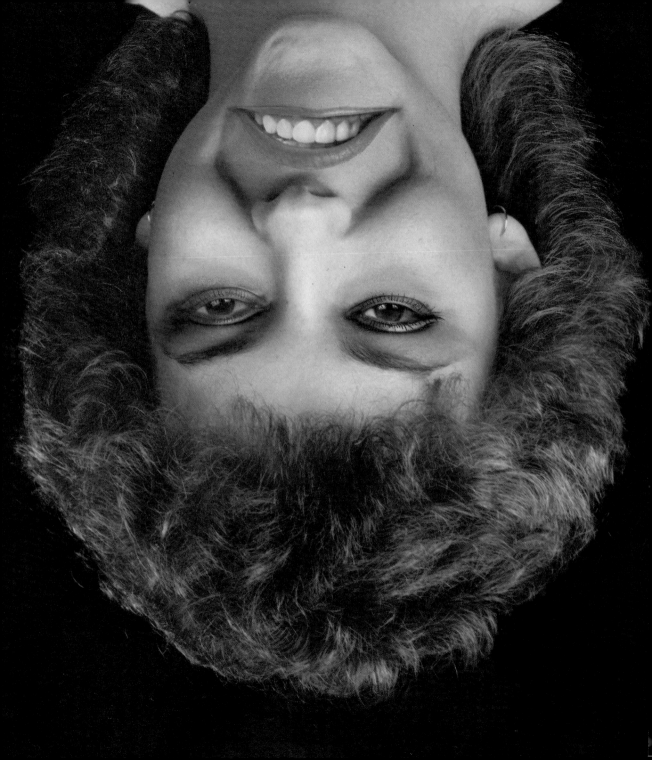

THE DECEPTIVE SMILE

To discover why this face appears strange, turn it upside down. Our eyes and brain are tricked by previous experience. The mouth and eyes have been left the right way up; the rest of the face is upside down. We perceive the mouth and eyes separately and use them to determine facial expressions. It does not seem to matter if they are in an impossible orientation (*see chapter 3 on Seeing*).

A THEORY OF CONNECTIONS

Like Broca, Wernicke did much more than simply identify an area on the left side of the brain which was concerned with language, and describe the problems of language which arose from its damage. Wernicke contributed a theory which explained our use of language by suggesting connections between areas of the brain, including Broca's area and Wernicke's area. These two areas are reasonably close together, and their proximity is no accident. Until a hundred years ago the vast majority of people were illiterate, and for them language was something which came in through their ears and out through their mouths.

Wernicke's area is located very near the area where sounds are deciphered by the brain. Broca's area, on the other hand, is just in front of the part which controls movements of the face, lips, tongue and other speech organs. It was therefore reasonable for Wernicke to assume that sounds pass through the ear into the brain, then to Wernicke's area, then through a 'telephone line', the *arcuate fasciculus*, to Broca's area, which further processes the information and passes it back to the region concerned with the muscular control of the speech organs, enabling words and sentences to be formed by the mouth and tongue. Geschwind believes that most language can be explained in terms of connections of this kind between brain areas. When a word is read, the visual stimulus is transmitted from other brain areas to Wernicke's area, where its heard form is produced. Then it goes through the same pathways as a heard word. Writing a word to dictation, on the other hand, requires the information to be passed from Wernicke's area, where the sounds are processed, to a visual area, where the sounds are translated into visual form preparatory to writing. This plan or model of the language system is not accepted by all neurologists. But it does certainly enable Professor Geschwind to make uncannily accurate diagnoses of brain damage by using only observations of the particular form of language defect he encounters in the particular patient. In many cases, it has been possible to confirm his diagnosis after the death of the patient by post mortem examination of his or her brain.

Happily, Charles Landry's brain is not yet available for post mortem examination. But the character of his language disability, and its improvement in the years since his stroke, has enabled Geschwind to assess his brain damage. What, asked Geschwind, was the first word Charles spoke after his stroke? 'I couldn't speak. Then I said "nurkle".' He smiled and shrugged his shoulders, as bewildered as his hearers. Now, though his speech is faltering, he can hold his own in one of Geschwind's searching examinations. Does he have damage in Broca's area, or can we locate the problem in Wernicke's area?

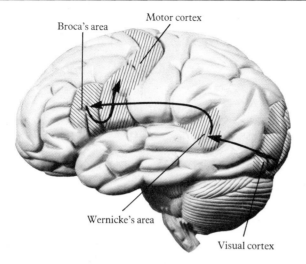

Broca's area
Motor cortex
Wernicke's area
Visual cortex

ROUTES FOR READING ALOUD
Words on this page are detected by the eyes which send appropriate signals along the optic nerves, eventually reaching the visual cortex at the back of the brain, to be analyzed as visual patterns. Then on to Wernicke's area for linguistic analysis, forward to Broca's area and then to the motor cortex for articulation. (Presumably silent reading involves all but the final stage.)

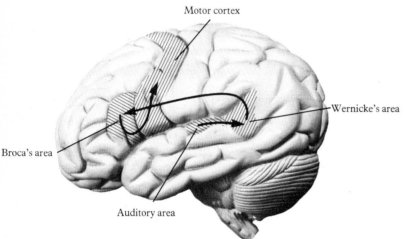

Motor cortex
Wernicke's area
Broca's area
Auditory area

ROUTES FOR REPETITION
Carl Wernicke proposed that a word heard in either ear travelled, as nerve impulses, to the auditory cortex for initial deciphering of the sounds. The signals then travelled to Wernicke's area, in the left hemisphere, for more analysis, then to Broca's area for conversion back into a form suitable for speech, and then on to that part of the motor cortex which controls movements of the mouth and tongue for speech.

A DIAGNOSIS

As is clear to the careful listener, Charles Landry does not speak like a patient with obvious damage in Broca's area, because he does not leave out the little words, the 'ifs', the 'ands', the 'buts' and the 'tos'. He does not leave out the endings, such as 's' in the possessive or the plural. His speech does not have the 'telegrammic' quality of Broca's aphasia. When Mr Landry speaks he may, like many such patients, have tremendous difficulty starting to speak, but his sentences are usually grammatically correct.

So Charles Landry's damage does not seem to be a simple destruction of Broca's area. In the following conversation, Geschwind probes further to discover exactly what deduction Landry's language problems may lead him towards.

GESCHWIND: Do you ever have any trouble with understanding what I say?

GESCHWIND: Well, let's just see. Now suppose you
wanted to communicate with a person who was in a
distant city, what apparatus would you utilize?

LANDRY: Telephone.

GESCHWIND: Very good. I deliberately made that a sort
of curious sentence. Now, let me ask you, do dogs fly?

LANDRY: No.

GESCHWIND: Do submarines usually fly?

LANDRY: No.

GESCHWIND: Can a Zeppelin fly?

LANDRY: Yes.

Charles Landry answered clearly, and for him, rapidly to each of
Geschwind's questions, and up to this point it is not possible to
decide whether he really has language difficulties. That was
resolved very quickly when Norman Geschwind began to examine
his understanding of a particular type of sentence.

The following exchange is a pointer to the precise position of
the damage in his brain.

GESCHWIND: Do you know what a leopard is?

LANDRY: Yes.

GESCHWIND: Do you know what a lion is?

LANDRY: Yes.

GESCHWIND: OK. A leopard was killed by the lion.
Which animal died?

LANDRY: I don't know.

GESCHWIND: That's hard is it?

LANDRY: I don't know . . . what animal died. . . . I don't
know.

Professor Geschwind explains that such failure has to be an error in
understanding grammar. If the 'grammatical' words are removed
then a normal person would have the same problem. It would be
rather like hearing: Buzz leopard buzz killed buzz lion. So that
the small grammatical words, particularly 'by' in this case, pose a
problem to Mr Landry. The same applies to the endings:

GESCHWIND: If I said to you 'That's my uncle's sister',
would that be a man or a woman?

LANDRY: I don't know, because . . . I don't know.

A tray was then produced with several objects on it, a pen, a pencil, a
watch, a coin. Geschwind asked him to touch the pencil with the
pen. Charles Landry hesitated, then picked up the pencil, hesitated
again, then touched the pen with it. It was clear that he had guessed
at the meaning of the sentence, but that he had no idea what the

'little words' added to the meaning. It is as if he had heard 'touch pencil pen' with meaningless sounds in the positions of 'the' and 'with the'. Geschwind followed this with one of his wry flights of fancy. 'Anybody who studied Latin could appreciate what it would be like to take a Latin sentence and remove all the endings from the words. You would have no idea what was being said, and I presume that in ancient Rome that's the way people with damage in Broca's area spoke.' In his thousands of examinations of Americans with Broca's area damage Geschwind very frequently finds this special kind of difficulty in *understanding* the 'little words'. He finds it also in spontaneous speech: such patients leave out the little words, and when asked to repeat sentences they also leave out the 'little words'. So in most patients the failure is in all three aspects of spoken language, understanding, spontaneous speech, and repetition. Mr Landry is so perplexing because he does not have these errors in spontaneous speech or in repetition, but in comprehension he has the difficulty in a most dramatic fashion, which makes him very much out of the ordinary.

What, then, was the site of Charles Landry's brain damage? While he showed some of the typical symptoms of the patient with damage in Broca's area, he showed none of the signs that the neurologist would take to indicate damage in Wernicke's area. Yet clearly his speech, and especially his understanding, were considerably impaired. Even if Geschwind had not known of his previous history he would have guessed that the damage had been in Broca's area, that the typical Broca's aphasia symptoms would have shown up sharply immediately after the stroke; but that in the intervening period some form of recovery of language had taken place. Geschwind knew that there were signs of paralysis in Charles's right side, and the right side of his face was also partially paralysed, which pointed unequivocally to damage in a specific area, the lower end of the motor cortex on the left side. And Broca's area is not far away from there. Add to that the difficulty Landry has with grammar and with comprehension of sentences using small words, and all the evidence suggests damage somewhere in the region of Broca's area.

PICTURES OF THE BRAIN

Not long before this examination, Charles Landry had his brain scanned by Computerized Axial Tomography, the technique used for the original Broca brain specimen. There was a very obvious area of damage on the left side, but Broca's area itself was spared because the damage was not on the surface but in the depths of the brain. That explains the right side paralysis, because the motor cortex sends out fibres which descend towards the lower part of the brain and the spinal cord, and those fibres have been cut off by the damage. In addition groups of cells lying deeply in the brain have been destroyed, particularly the cells that make up the putamen.

The putamen is part of the basal ganglia, which we know to be involved in both the control of movement and emotions (see Chapter 4 on movement). Taken with the damage to fibres involved in movement, running down from the motor cortex to the spinal cord, this might suggest that in Charles Landry's case the language deficit is caused by damage to the system controlling movement, the motor system. But this is quite certainly too simple an interpretation. At the moment Geschwind admits that there is no adequate knowledge of the mechanism of these areas which could explain how damage to them disrupts Charles Landry's language abilities. But our current ignorance of the detailed mechanisms is not, in Geschwind's view, a reason for not pursuing such investigations.

He believes that to succeed in treating aphasias well requires knowledge of how language is organized in the brain. Once that is obtained and it is known exactly where the damage is, and what the chemical substances involved are, and what the connections within the brain are, then doctors should be able to alter that system and bring in areas of undamaged brain to restore language. The basic concept is no different from that used to treat diabetes or high blood pressure or any disease.

How the Brain Recovers Skills

It is clear that Charles Landry's language capabilities have improved very substantially, despite our present ignorance, since that first word 'nurkle'. Is there any understanding of how his brain has coped so much better with language than in those first, post-stroke, days? Geschwind is sure that it is not the growth of new nerve cells, because adults just cannot grow new ones. Nor is it a reduction in the swelling round the original damage, because that disappears in two or three weeks. So Mr Landry's recovery must be either the result of new learning somewhere in the brain, or the re-activation of learning which was there before but was not available. It may even be a result of some kind of re-organization of the chemistry of the brain which allows some cells to fire which were suppressed. Geschwind does not know the answer. However, as mentioned above, when damage occurs before the age of eight on the left side the child's recovery of language is excellent or even perfect. Also, certain adults recover better than others. Left-handers seem to recover better from the damage to language areas than right-handers, fitting in with the fact that left-handers have a much less localized kind of brain and their language ability seems to be distributed much more diffusely.

An examination of Charles Landry's problems, therefore, contributes to our understanding of the language areas in the brain, and the pathways between them. We shall see later in the chapter how Geschwind applies his technique to a second case of language disability.

MAPPING THE NORMAL BRAIN

It would obviously be easier to find out how a telephone system works by looking at a plan of the system than by tracing the wires in the system after one of them has broken, and deducing how the system operates from that evidence. In the same way, there are inherent problems in trying to understand the language system by examining patients whose system has been damaged. While we can certainly say that damage in Broca's area, and in Wernicke's area, does lead to rather specific defects in language, and can trace some other defects that occur because of damage to other areas or structures in the brain, we still do not have a full picture of the system as a whole. Already, from Professor Geschwind's examination of Charles Landry, we can see that the system is too complicated for that. We need to know exactly which areas and connections are used in the normal production of language, but until recently there has been no way of establishing which parts of the brain are active during the production of language.

Earlier in this chapter we described the computerized X-rays which can show areas of damage at different levels in the brain more effectively than conventional X-rays. But these are static pictures, and we need a way of showing particular areas when the brain is at work. Now it is possible to do this with an apparatus known as the Positron Emission Tomograph, or PET scan, which maps the brain's metabolism of food. The brain is a fierce consumer of sugar, in the form of glucose. If it is supplied with a special form of glucose which cannot be broken down and turned into food, but which is radio-active, then the radio-active 'glucose' will show up for a time in those brain areas which are absorbing it and trying to utilize it as

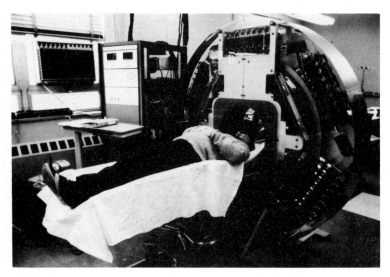

SCANNING THE ACTIVE BRAIN
In this new technique, Positron Emission Tomography, the brain concentrates a radioactive chemical in the regions most active during a task, and the machine measures radioactivity as positron emissions. Like the computerized X-ray, PET scans can also show regions of brain damage where little radioactivity is retained by the dead tissue.

food. Thus active areas are shown in one colour, shading off to relatively inert areas in another colour.

A psychologist at the University of Pennsylvania, Ruben Gur, volunteered to use the PET scan to show which parts of his brain were made active during a verbal task. The specially-prepared radio-active glucose has a half-life of only four hours, and is made at a nuclear research laboratory two hundred miles from Philadelphia; so it has to be rushed by air to the PET scan laboratory otherwise the radio-activity would already be too low when it arrived.

Dr Gur does not speak during the exercise, because that would cause the parts of the brain concerned with the movement of his mouth and jaw to 'light up': that is, to use more glucose. So his colleagues set him a verbal task in which he has to find out the relationship between words. This task should light up those areas of his brain which are involved in language, but not involved specifically in the action of speech.

Curiously enough, the PET scan on Ruben Gur showed that wide areas of the brain, certainly not limited to the left-hand side, were involved in the processing of language. This by no means invalidates Geschwind's theory of localization. It points, rather, to the involvement of many other brain areas which are concerned with faculties that are inevitably associated with language. The visual areas, and the auditory areas, may become involved because of visual or verbal associations. And memory, in which we believe the hippocampus and neighbouring areas are involved, must also be needed for language ability. If memory is involved, it is likely that large areas of the cortex will become active, since there may be dispersal of memory stores over the whole cortex (see Chapter 1 on memory). It should not be surprising that so far-reaching a human characteristic as language should involve much of the warp and weft of the brain, much of what the pioneer physiologist, Sherrington,

PATTERNS OF BRAIN ACTIVITY
The machine seen opposite produces images like these which scientists can use to trace activity in various parts of the brain. Different areas of the brain are active depending on what the person is doing (*see frontispiece*).

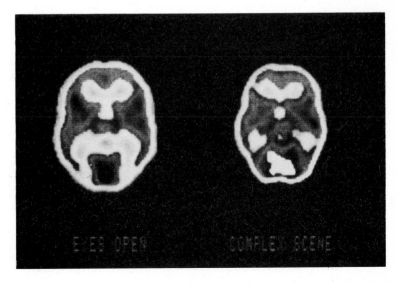

described as 'an enchanted loom'. The brain is so complex in its internal connections that it would be presumptuous, in our present state of knowledge, to suggest that we can limit the astonishing faculty of language to only a few areas of tissue.

Patients Who Write, but Cannot Read

The connection between speaking, reading and writing must also be considered in any study of language. It is often the case, as it is with Charles Landry, that disorders of spoken language will be accompanied also with reading problems. For example, Charles could not read aloud the sentence 'Are there four of us in here?', although he could understand its meaning. There are more striking, and at first sight more puzzling cases. Many neurologists have reported cases of pure alexia without agraphia. This is neurologists' language for the problem of being able to write but not able to read. So a person may write an answer to a question quite correctly, but not be able to read it back: even though he can see it. These strange, but presumably in real life very sad, cases have damage in areas further back in the brain than Broca's or Wernicke's area. In these rare cases the visual cortex at the back of the brain on the left is destroyed, and as a result the patient can perceive written material only using the right visual region. For this material to be interpreted as language, it must be relayed to the language areas on the left side, via part of the corpus callosum, the great bundle of fibres which joins the left cerebral hemisphere to the right hemisphere. These cases have damage there, to the specific part of the corpus callosum at the back, which transfers information from the visual areas to language areas. This can no longer take place, so information about words remains in the right hemisphere, which cannot comprehend them. So this bizarre condition can be explained purely in terms of severed telephone lines within the brain.

Cases in which the left visual cortex has been destroyed, but the corpus callosum has not been injured do not result in people with 'alexia without agraphia'. Such patients' ability both to write and read is explained by the preservation of the corpus callosum, which can now pass information from the right hemisphere to the language left. In cases where the whole of the corpus callosum has been cut or otherwise destroyed, many other very striking symptoms have been observed and these are examined in detail in Chapter 7. It is another interesting sidelight on the history of neurology that, although curious symptoms following damage to the corpus callosum were reported as early as 1892, and continued to be of interest in Germany and France, the British and American view was that destruction of the corpus callosum appeared to cause no problem. This failure to reach the correct conclusions from the evidence persisted until 1960, supported by reports in early 1940 that destruction of the corpus callosum produced no apparent effects in humans or animals. The subsequent change of view resulted directly from the work of Roger Sperry (for which he received the Nobel Prize in 1981), and from the interest of neurologists, chief among them Norman Geschwind, attempting to explain the symptoms of their patients in simple and precise ways related to our knowledge of the brain.

LANGUAGE, AND THE RIGHT HEMISPHERE

Although there is not much doubt that the left hemisphere dominates our faculty of language, the contribution of the right hemisphere cannot be altogether discounted. The next case we encountered, in England this time, demonstrated some further peculiarities in the comprehension of language which may be explained by some activity, or lack of it, in the right hemisphere.

This time, the study was being done by psychologists, not neurologists, and they were from the Medical Research Council's Applied Psychology Unit at Cambridge. The gentleman who was the subject of the psychologists' interest was Mr Percy Ward, a retired local government official, born in 1908, who had a stroke in 1965. He appears to be a sufferer from Broca's aphasia, in a more extreme form than Charles Landry, so that his speech is impaired, though adequate for rather limited conversational purposes. He has kept his sense of humour and, like Mr Landry, puts a lot of effort into improving his language. Although he is often tired and frustrated he never gives up. Mr Ward is a celebrated case of a rather newly labelled disability, 'deep dyslexia'. The name was coined only in 1971, and it is rather different from the dyslexia we normally think of when we hear the term, often applied to children who cannot read properly. Mr Ward has lost nearly all the language areas in his left hemisphere. He is an engaging and good-tempered person, who obviously thoroughly enjoys the visits of Canadian psychologist, Karalyn Patterson, from the Applied Psychology Unit.

Dr Patterson showed Mr Ward a series of cards on which words were printed. His responses demonstrated the range of his abilities and strange disabilities. He was able to read 'mile', 'flood', 'yacht', 'borough', 'cough', 'wigwam' and many more with no errors and as quickly as a healthy individual. He could even distinguish between 'borough' and 'cough'. Then Dr Patterson showed Mr Ward a card with the word 'duel' on it.

MR WARD: Er, er, sword, or spear, or, er, sword.
KARALYN PATTERSON: Is it sword?
MR WARD: Raper, raper, er, rapier.
KARALYN PATTERSON: Rapier, is that it?
MR WARD: Rapier.
KARALYN PATTERSON: OK.

He then read 'corner', 'dancing', 'danger' with no errors. Then another card which puzzled Mr Ward. The word printed on it was 'hermit'.

>MR WARD: . . . Oh yes. . . . Monk, monk.
>KARALYN PATTERSON: Well, you tell me, is it monk?
>MR WARD: No, no, monk, no. Oh dear. . . . Recluse.
>KARALYN PATTERSON: Is it recluse?
>MR WARD: Recluse.
>KARALYN PATTERSON: OK, you're happy with that.

Evidently, somewhere in Mr Ward's brain there was a mechanism which recognized the words 'duel' and 'hermit' but which, for some reason, was unable to repeat them. Yet Mr Ward was able to produce, quite accurately, words which reflected the associations of the word 'duel'. In the case of 'hermit' he sought about for the most appropriate word, rejecting 'monk', but eventually agreeing that the sophisticated response 'recluse' was close enough.

The response of Mr Ward and of other so-called deep dyslexics to the tests suggests an explanation to Karalyn Patterson and other psychologists. The explanation is, remember, a psychologist's explanation and not a neurologist's. Psychologists certainly pay attention to the brain, its areas and its connections, but they are more concerned with working out the logic of particular symptoms such as deep dyslexia. Not all psychologists, and certainly few neurologists, would agree with the explanation.

In deep dyslexia, the argument runs, whatever the graphic form of a word, whether it is hand-written, or printed in any sort of type, the brain recognizes it as a particular word: so the brain must, argue the psychologists, contain a system for identifying words. They call it, reasonably enough, a word identifier. Wherever this word identifier may be in the brain, further processing takes place which links up the signals from it to other related elements in the brain, which assign a 'meaning' to the word. Referred to further systems, those signals are processed and converted into a form which is finally spoken aloud. This final processing probably takes place, the psychologists agree, in Broca's area. Somewhere in this system, Mr Ward's disability can be explained.

Normal people also have the ability to read words that they have not encountered before and to pronounce them, doing it letter by letter. That can be tested directly in deep dyslexia. Dr Patterson showed Mr Ward a card on which was written the three letters H, E and B. Percy Ward looked at the card.

>MR WARD: Sorry.
>KARALYN PATTERSON: Is it a word?
>MR WARD: No.
>KARALYN PATTERSON: No. But even though it's not a

word it's a collection of letters that could be pronounced. You could say these aloud.
MR WARD: Er, hod, hod.

He looked at Karalyn Patterson and smiled. 'Me. . . . Help!' he said.

KARALYN PATTERSON: Yes, it looks something like
help but have you any idea what that set of letters would
sound like if you pronounced it?
MR WARD: Sorry, no.

A PSYCHOLOGICAL EXPLANATION

Dr Patterson explained the results of her tests in the terms of the
psychological theory. Obviously Mr Ward cannot convert letters
into sounds, that ability is missing. But he can see and work out the
shapes of the letters as quickly as anybody else. The 'word
identifier' is also working properly, because he knows that 'heb' and
other nonsense strings of letters are not words. He also connects
words with what the psychologists call 'meaning', because when he
looks at 'duel' and says 'sword' or 'rapier', there is a close
connection between our associations with 'sword' and Mr Ward's
responses. He clearly lacks the ability to get from these associations
to the correct pronunciation.

However, 'duel' and 'hermit' are both nouns, and when Mr
Ward is asked to read words with other grammatical functions he
often fails. For example, he cannot read 'to' or 'if' despite many
valiant attempts, but if there is some concrete or even sensory
association he may read correctly or get close. He read 'her' as 'she'
and 'yours' as 'you', and could read 'merry'. Clearly he has the
ability to understand the use of many, but by no means all words,
and he does have as much difficulty understanding the 'little words'
as Charles Landry. Being a Broca's aphasic, Mr Ward of course not
only has trouble understanding them but using them too.

Psychologists like Karalyn Patterson are anxious to understand the various processes of language, and if possible to separate
one from another. We see this to be the case in the chapter on
memory, and with language the proposition is the same: if there are
different processes happening in the 'mind', then it may be
reasonable to assume that there are different areas of the brain
dealing with these processes. If this is the case, then in normal
reading we use different processes, and perhaps different parts of
the brain, for reading words by their visual characteristics and for
reading words by sounding out the letters to ourselves. The
hypothesis seems to be supported by evidence other than that from
the group of deep dyslexics studied by Karalyn Patterson and her
colleagues. For example, there is a case of a professor of philosophy
in France who suffered extensive brain damage following a stroke.

At first he appeared to have lost the ability to read, but it became apparent after a few months of testing that not only did he show similar ability in reading to Mr Ward but that he could also 'speed read' which one would not have expected in a brain-damaged patient. The hypothesis is that in the case of the professor, as in the case of Mr Ward, the processes for recognizing a whole word and assigning it 'meaning' still worked, whereas the slower process of identifying a word and using it through assembling its component letters and sounds did not work. Other evidence comes from Japan. Japanese writing is a combination of Kana (in which symbols are used to represent separate syllables) and Kanji, derived from Chinese writing and therefore pictographic, in which a single complex symbol is used to represent a whole word. Japanese patients with aphasia may be able to read only Kana writing or only Kanji writing: again, this seems to support the idea that different processes are used for reading words visually and reading words by sounding them out, letter by letter, or syllable by syllable. If the theory is correct it of course carries certain implications about our normal method of reading, and about our methods of teaching children to read. The 'look and say' approach may be used by the normal brain as well as the 'ABC' approach. The theory may eventually help speech therapists to re-train stroke patients.

In the PET scan large areas of the brain, and not only those on the left, seemed to be involved in processing language, though not in speech. Dr Patterson also believes that in deep dyslexia we may be seeing a language capability in the right hemisphere being used to overcome a disability. The right hemisphere may analyse a word visually, recognize it as a word, and understand its 'meaning', but has only a very limited ability actually to produce speech. Vicki and Paul, two split brain patients that we described in Chapter 7, do appear to have some ability to write words using their right hemisphere. They are the only split brain patients investigated so far who have this ability.

A NEUROLOGICAL EXPLANATION

Norman Geschwind would certainly agree that the right hemisphere does not produce speech, at least in the case of a normal adult whose left hemisphere has been extensively damaged in the language areas. But he does not agree with the psychological theory advanced by Dr Patterson. His approach is rather different, because he has seen the same pattern of errors when aphasic patients heard words, rather than read them. For example, when asked to repeat 'President' they would say 'Reagan'. He believes that these patients are doing exactly the same thing as the deep dyslexics and, in addition, when they read they also have more trouble with the 'small' words. So the abilities that are missing may not be connected solely with reading, but with the handling of words by the brain in

NORMAL AND ABNORMAL READING

To read the word 'tree' aloud a normal individual transfers information from the eyes to the visual cortex on both sides. Then analysis takes place in Wernicke's and Broca's areas on the left. If someone suffering from deep dyslexia, like Mr Ward, tries to read the word 'tree', one possible explanation for his errors is that the signals are blocked by damage in the left hemisphere of his brain. He then transfers the signals to the right side, but because he cannot deal with language there in the normal way, they summon up non-verbal associations instead, such as the memories of wood, branch or orchard. By the time the information returns to the left hemisphere for conversion back to speech, the original word has changed.

any form. He thinks that the damage prevents correct repetition because the patient cannot transfer the heard word from Wernicke's area forward to Broca's area, due to damage in between, so he learns to use alternative routes. For example, somebody being given a word like 'tree' might transfer it from the left hemisphere over to the right hemisphere where it might arouse an association. Then he might pass that association forward to another location in the right hemisphere and somehow use a long detour to get to the speech area in the left hemisphere. But by then the word would be in a non-verbal form: it might be a visual memory, for example, and what might be spoken could be a word like 'orchard'. That could occur regardless of whether the word had originally been read or heard, or even if it was a picture or something that the patient had held in his hand.

Norman Geschwind is at pains not to discount the worth of the work done on deep dyslexia. He thinks that its great value is that it has posed a problem that both linguists and neurologists keep avoiding. He assumes that the function of language is to give information about the world. Little is known about how it does this and deep dyslexia may force scientists to think about how language does come into the brain and so permits us to match what goes on inside the brain to what is going on outside in the real world.

We all take our capacity for language for granted. It is as natural as breathing or eating or sleeping. It is only when something

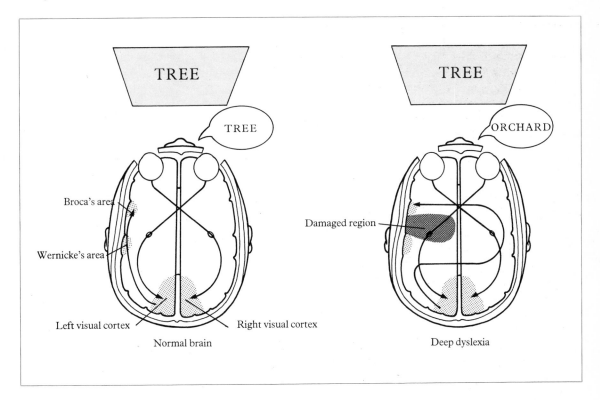

Broca's area

Wernicke's area

Damaged region

Left visual cortex   Right visual cortex

Normal brain   Deep dyslexia

goes wrong, perhaps when someone suffers a stroke, like Charles Landry, that our brain's effortless coping with the miraculous processes of understanding or speaking or reading is called into question. Somewhere inside Charles Landry's head, he still seems to understand even the complicated legal phraseology of the documents he used to use in his law practice. But he cannot get that understanding out of his brain and into his speech to make the link between understanding and conveying understanding which is necessary to him to communicate with anyone else. We asked him to read one of the laws of the State of Massachusetts to himself. He did so, and paraphrased it well, but could not read it aloud. One of the words which confused him was 'conceals'. He kept looking at it: 'Conceals . . . that this is mushy gush, because conceals is . . . it's not conceals, it's anything. This is not conceals, you know, it's anything, it's chair, desk, table, but not conceals. So, it's a mystery. It's a mystery.'

Charles Landry is right. It is a mystery. We know an enormous amount about how the brain works, its electrical signals, its chemical modulators, its connections, its anatomy. But we are an enormous distance away from the goal to which all the neurologists and all the psychologists aspire. We are woefully inadequate at connecting our human abilities to the grey and white matter of our brains. The number of brain cells and their almost infinite number of interconnections is so overwhelming that it is almost impossible to conceive of a time when we will understand those so clearly that we can associate them with our own behaviour. That will only be possible when not only the psychologists and the neurologists can speak the same language, but when we can combine all the sciences that study the brain into one science. That is an enormous task. The amount of data produced by all the brain sciences is already vast, and no one man can hope to read, let alone comprehend, all of it. Many people may even find that the attempt to reduce our own nature to the functioning of cells within the brain is distasteful, but Norman Geschwind is not one of them. His dedication to the prevention or treatment of brain damage is too deep seated for him to jib at abstract philosophical issues of that kind.

It's always curious to me that sometimes people come along and say, 'Well, this is a very bad way to look at things because it takes away the human quality of human beings. It makes people into some kind of mechanism.' And my response to that is that what is most humanizing is to free humans from those things which prevent them from living as humans. Now I don't see any great advantage for a patient to be forced to remain aphasic for twenty years of his life because we have no adequate means of treating that. I think that in practice it may well be possible to release stores of language which are present but unavailable. I cannot believe that by learning about the mechanism of how and where language is stored and being able to use that knowledge to treat patients, that we would not be increasing human freedom rather than diminishing it. As a result I can't take seriously at all the arguments that looking at people in this way is somehow making them more into machines and less human.

The notion of the human as a machine is not a simple one, as we shall discover in later chapters, nor is it a dehumanizing one. In the next three we shall examine more ancient faculties than language, faculties we share with far simpler creatures than ourselves. Without these faculties that developed far back in evolution we could never have developed to speak and understand language; but, because they are more primitive they are, in some ways at least, easier to describe and understand, more machine-like, perhaps. We may find it difficult to believe that we are biological machines; but the idea is not by any means useless as a way of understanding the functioning of our brains.

CHAPTER 3

SEEING

To enable humans to function in the world they need to take information from the senses. That is a necessary first step before acting on that information; so this chapter on seeing precedes the chapter on movement, input preceding output. Sight is the sense that must stand here to represent all five senses. And if we think of it as input, we are already using the terms applied to computers: input, information processing, output. This chapter will use the computer as more than an analogy, because brain science and computer science have developed together; some scientists believe that a computer can be used to represent, however crudely, some of the brain's functions. Those representations must be based on existing knowledge of the brain and of seeing and what it is for. The computer here is not being used to replace man's brain, but to understand it.

FROM EYE TO BRAIN

Our world is the world of our sight, of all our senses the most immediate and all embracing. But that world of reality is somehow created from pencils of light refracted through the crystalline lenses

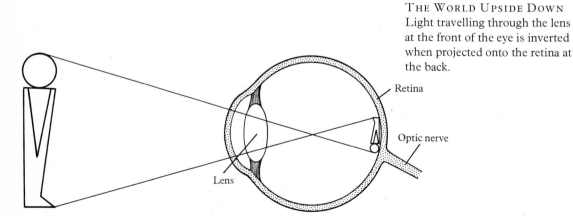

THE WORLD UPSIDE DOWN
Light travelling through the lens at the front of the eye is inverted when projected onto the retina at the back.

Retina

Optic nerve

Lens

PATHWAYS OF VISION

Each eye views both left and right sides of the visual field (as you can check by looking straight ahead, and closing first one eye, then the other). However, the brain receives left and right visual fields separately because of a cross-over where the optic nerves intersect at the optic chiasma. Signals from the *left* visual field of *both* eyes travel via the lateral geniculate body in the midbrain to the *right* visual cortex where seeing really begins. Conversely, the left visual cortex receives signals from the right visual field.

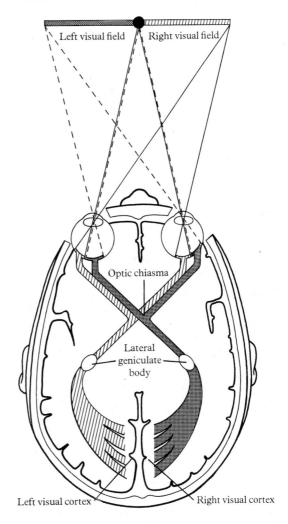

Left visual field   Right visual field

Optic chiasma

Lateral geniculate body

Left visual cortex   Right visual cortex

of our eyes. As the lens on a camera focuses an image on to the sensitive emulsion of the film, the lens of our eye focuses a scene on to the sensitive cells of the retina that curves round the back of the eyeball. From the retina a soft twisting cable of nerves carries signals back to our brains, and it is in our brains that reality, the world outside, the seen world, the three-dimensional world, takes shape. It is created therefore from the firing of nerves: seeing is an illusion. There are no pictures inside our heads.

The house-fly can see the descending fly swat and take evasive action in a split second, and the eagle can see a shrew running among grasses hundreds of feet below him. We see the world more clearly than the fly, but without the precision of the gliding eagle. Yet we can perceive minute variations in the shape of a face, and recognize one among tens of thousands. We can discriminate between the texture of mink fur and rabbit fur, between glass and diamond, between shades of colour that vary by only the minutest degree. But the vision of all animals, including ourselves, is intended for the same purposes, to see an object and decide what to do about it: whether to run away from it or eat it. How do our brains interpret the events in the world of sight? It is difficult to imagine how it could be done unless there are pictures in our heads.

VISION, AND THE MIND OF THE ARTIST

One man who believes that he does indeed have pictures in his head is the artist Anthony Green RA, yet he is faced with a paradox. He knows, too, that all that is really inside his head is a mass of grey and white nerve cells, and that the scientific viewpoint is that there are no pictures. 'Tripe!' says he. 'I've got pictures inside my head and I suspect you've got some in yours as well. I can see them, just as you can see them. You can remember your living room. Shut your eyes and look at it . . . look at your dining room. Shut your eyes and remember. It's there in pictures!'

Anthony Green's paintings are detailed reconstructions of scenes from his memories. They are not exactly realistic; no one would think an Anthony Green chair was a real chair, and try to sit on it. But the paintings have an immediate quality which somehow rings very true, and the painter distorts and manipulates perspective and form to create this immediacy for his 'memory pictures', as he calls them. He paints, not from models, but from his memories. His description of the processes he goes through to arrive at the finished picture is curiously close to the way scientists are beginning to think about vision, as we shall see later.

Scientists can only make progress by assuming that there are no pictures in our heads and their evidence comes from several directions. One is from the blind.

THE VISION OF THE BLIND

If we could imagine seeing without using our eyes, but by using a few square inches of skin, would it then be possible to describe what we 'saw' as pictures? This may appear to be a rather abstract philosophical experiment; but it has really been performed by blind people. One such was Gerard Guarniero, who has been blind from birth. To give himself some experience of a sense he has never had, Dr Guarniero went to San Francisco, to the Smith-Kettlewell Institute of Visual Sciences, to experiment with a device which gives him vision. The device goes under the name of the Tactile Visual Substitution System, or TVSS for short.

The system consists of a television camera linked to a rectangular mosaic of pins, 400 in number, which vibrate sixty times a second. Each pin covers a small area of the TV camera's field of view and only vibrates if that part of the field is light. The pins thus transmit the signal 'light' or 'dark' to a small area of the

experimental subject's back. The equipment is therefore convert-
ing a visual image into a tactile image, registering on the sense
receptors of the skin. It is coarse and limited when compared to true
vision, but Guarniero's comments on it are revealing.

> When I first started using it, it felt as if the images that
> the television camera was picking up were on my skin.
> But afterwards, the things I was seeing with the system
> really didn't feel as if they were on my skin any more. To
> give you an analogy, it's like when you are looking at
> something, you don't really see the object *in your eye*, or
> when you're listening to something, you really don't
> hear it *in your ear*; it's only when you're touching
> something that you appear to feel it on your skin, and the
> sensations that one gets through using the system don't
> feel as if they're *on the skin* any more after you use it for a
> while. I really can't convey the quality of the experience,
> and of course I really don't know what seeing would feel
> like. But it didn't feel as if it was on the skin, it felt as if it
> was somewhere in two-dimensional space of some sort
> that I was 'seeing' the objects. I think both vision and the
> TVSS in a sense take you outside of yourself, they carry
> you beyond yourself to the object.

Guarniero found a number of problems when he first started to use
the system. The first was that when he moved his head (to which the
camera was attached) the object appeared to move in the opposite
direction. This was at first unsettling, and he had to come to terms
with it, just as we sighted people already have. He also found that it
was difficult to make a correlation between the objects he was given
to look at – such things as watering cans, vases of artificial flowers,
toy horses and telephones – and the way they felt when he was asked
to handle them and examine them by touch. But he soon became
adept at reconciling the tactile and visual stimuli of specific objects.
At this stage a new camera was introduced, hand-held and fitted
with a zoom lens. This introduced a further problem, because if he
used the zoom it was difficult for Guarniero to judge the relative size
of different objects. As he continued to practise, however, he found
that the zoom could be used to investigate details of the object in
close-up. Of course, the detail was not very finely resolved, since the
system gave Guarniero only 400 black or white points – much as if a
television picture was composed of only twenty lines instead of 625.
    Next, Guarniero attempted to use the system to judge relative
distances between objects. To do this, he used some of the clues
sighted people use: for instance, if we see two similar objects, the
smaller will be likely to be the further away; or, when two objects are
viewed from above, the further away will appear higher in the visual
field. As the session went on, Guarniero said that he stopped

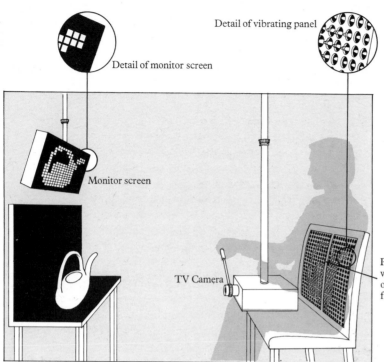

Detail of monitor screen

Detail of vibrating panel

Monitor screen

TV Camera

Panel of pins
which vibrate
on instruction
from TV camera.

SEEING ON THE SKIN

The apparatus used by the blind philosopher Guarniero to 'see' was a black and white TV camera which fed an array of blunt vibrating pins against the backs of sightless subjects. A pin would vibrate when light hit the appropriate part of the camera's field of view. He picked out details by zooming and panning the camera. To Dr Guarniero the pins did not feel as if they were on his back, but 'out there' ahead of him.

making conscious deliberations about the distance between objects, and was able to make judgements more instantaneously, as would a sighted person. He went on to judge the orientation of objects – which way the spout of the watering can or the head of the horse was facing. Perhaps his most unexpected experience was with a candle. 'I never knew that a flame had a definite shape, and I found the whole idea of watching a flame move extremely fascinating. If you go to examine a flame tactually all you feel is heat, and if it's hot enough of course you take your hands away, and you can't examine the shape of the flame.' One of the limitations of the system is that it is not stereoscopic, that the user sees (or feels) a picture only in two dimensions, making it difficult to recognize an irregularly shaped object if it is seen from more than one point of view. But when Guarniero was also given a turntable which he could control himself, he was able to rotate the objects and provide himself with some idea of the overall shape of a three-dimensional object.

Guarniero recognizes the difficulty he has in describing his experience with the TVSS. He uses the word 'see' but he cannot know that he is using it accurately. All he does know is that the experience he has from using the device is qualitatively different from the experience of touching an object and exploring it only by touch. He knows too that the information provided by the device first reaches the area in his brain normally concerned with touch, in the sensory strip of the cerebral cortex. Beyond this point, of course, the information may be treated in exactly the same way and by the same parts of the brain used for vision. But one thing is sure: no pictures reach his brain. Guarniero is therefore convinced of one thing. 'If there were pictures in the head, you would need somebody inside your head to look at the pictures, and that seems not to be the case. There is no one else inside your head looking at the pictures. Who could there be?'

There is no answer to that question, but one's response is to ask, 'What is there in the head then?' The new theory of vision now emerging goes some way to answering that. It begins with the idea that vision evolved to provide us human animals with information about the world so that we could function and thrive in it. If that is the case, seeing must be a process of matching: matching the external world with our internal one: watching and combining information coming in through each of the senses with the programmes in our brains that affect movement so that we can see, decide, and then move to suit the circumstances. That idea was tested by a series of experiments started eighty years ago, which we decided to try to repeat.

An Experiment with Vision and Perception

Towards the end of the nineteenth century, early days in the science of psychology, some of the keenest discussions about the psychology of vision centred around the question of how humans perceive upright objects. One school held that we only perceive objects as being the 'right way up' if their image is inverted. (The lens of the eye projects an upside-down image on to the back screen or retina, just like a camera lens.) This apparently paradoxical theory was explored by George M. Stratton of the University of California, in one of those alarming experiments which scientists in the nineteenth century performed on themselves. Stratton decided that he would make himself an apparatus which would turn the world upside down and, of course, would turn its image the right way up on his retina. In its final form the apparatus was an 8-inch-long tube mounted vertically over one eye and enclosed in plaster which Stratton had cast to the exact contours of his face. The other eye was blindfolded. The tube contained a set of lenses which would invert Stratton's image of the world. He wore it for eighty-seven hours over the period of a week, replacing it with a blindfold while he slept so that he would not be tempted to peek at the world in its normal orientation. Stratton's world was not only inverted, but left and right were reversed, as if in a mirror.

We decided to re-enact Stratton's experiment. A young art student, Susannah Fiennes, agreed to wear inverting spectacles for a week, and to report on her results to us. Neither she nor we realized how demanding it would be. If there were pictures in Susannah's head, turning them upside down should profoundly

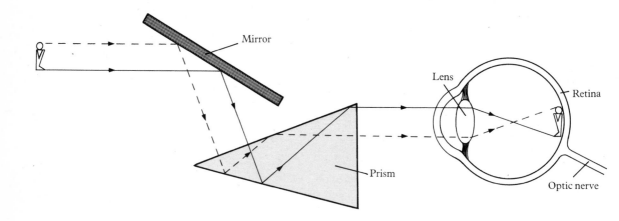

alter her experience and her perception of the real world. If, on the other hand, vision and perception are a process of the brain (and there are consequently no pictures in the head) the quality of her perception of the world should not be altered – or should it?

The glasses which Susannah wore were less horrific than Stratton's tube; they were not much larger than ordinary spectacles, because they used prisms instead of lenses, and she could use both eyes. They only inverted the world – left and right remained the same; but they did restrict her field of vision, giving her less peripheral vision, a sort of tunnel vision.

When Susannah put on her new glasses, her reaction on the homeward car journey was immediate and emotional. 'The cars are going upside down. They're going the wrong way. It's all going completely the wrong way to what you'd expect. It's really strange.'

After she had worn the spectacles for about an hour, she told us how she was feeling:

> When I was coming back in the car, I didn't feel as if it was any different, although I felt quite sick. In fact, looking at people in cars was quite normal, I didn't think they were upside down, and I just got adjusted to it, I think. But the difficult thing is just walking and being very disorientated, because how you feel is completely different to what you're doing. It's very confusing, I think. [Even at this point, Susannah's brain is beginning to make an interpretation of the world it sees.] As for things being upside down, it just doesn't feel like that at all because I know very well that I'm sitting here, and so I think my brain still knows that, so it's all right.

First of all, strange though things look, they are apparently not upside down: another nail in the coffin of the pictures in the head

INVERTING SPECTACLES
A system of mirrors and prisms which inverts the object before it reaches the eye, but the eye turns it again, so that it is upright on the retina. In the 19th century scientists experienced such bizarre effects with a similar system that their attitude to vision changed. But both to them and to a modern subject, Susannah Fiennes, the world did not seem upside down!

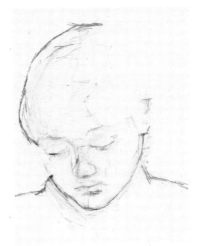

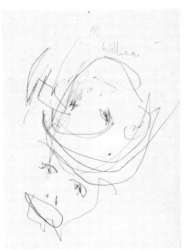

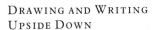

DRAWING AND WRITING UPSIDE DOWN

Susannah Fiennes, an art student, did the sketch of her brother on the left just before wearing her inverting spectacles. On the right is her attempt one day after putting them on. At this early stage she is not seeing in the true sense, merely responding to the pattern of light and shade.

After two days Susannah tried printing her name, first with her eyes closed (*top two versions*). Her brain was confused and sent some incorrect signals to her hand. She did the third version so that she could read it. The final attempt was to write correctly while looking.

idea. Secondly, the difficulties she has are with movement: matching vision with her muscles' movements.

Susannah had attempted to pour milk from a jug into a glass, one of George Stratton's tests on himself. She found this extremely difficult, since she could not judge the relative levels of jug and glass; when she thought she was raising the jug she was in fact lowering it. But she was determined, and the milk did get into the glass, with not too many drops split.

By the fourth day she could walk without difficulty, even with poise, from her bedroom into the sitting room. And the milk-jug test went smoothly. How was she feeling? 'Just fine, you know, there's no difference. I don't notice that things are upside down at all.'

George Stratton reported that during the first few nights when he went to bed wearing his blindfold he had imagined the world the right way up. Subsequently he began to feel that his night-time vision of the world was now upside down. Susannah felt the same thing. 'I'm now beginning to imagine things upside down, not just see them like that, so I suppose my brain is becoming more and more convinced, although I am still aware that it is not real.' This process went through various stages. After four days she was still able to write her name normally, but only if she closed her eyes and did not see her hand as it wrote. With eyes open she was able to write Susannah so that it appeared normal to her inverted vision, but that meant it was upside down for everyone else. It was still very difficult for her to write a normal 'upright' signature while watching her hand through the experimental spectacles; it came out half correct and half inverted. This is another example of the gradual matching of actions with visual perceptions which constitutes the process of seeing.

After a week her early problems seemed to have vanished. 'I can more or less do everything. I've been riding a bicycle, I can walk, I can run quite easily and go up and down the stairs and turn corners. . . . I can make cups of coffee and put on records. The only thing that's still quite difficult is eating and using a knife and fork.' Immediately after putting the spectacles on Susannah had felt more comfortable sitting still; now all the normal actions of everyday life had become much easier. And her subjective feelings had changed too. 'It's become more and more difficult to imagine myself standing upright or sitting down normally. I almost want to sit upside down because I can't quite imagine myself sitting normally.' Her experience supports the idea central to the new theory of seeing, that it is an active process to enable us to deal with the world.

When Susannah took off the spectacles after a week of wearing them continuously, and normal vision was restored, it was a revelation to her. 'There's no difference. That's what's so extraordinary. There's no difference at all. Perhaps because it's so familiar anyway, and I can just think back to what I knew it was anyway, but I can't think of it as any different now to what it was just last night.' Susannah had reverted to normal vision within a few minutes, with a feeling of considerable relief that the experiment was over.

The image on Susannah's retina had been turned round 180 degrees, and there was no doubt that her *method* of seeing had changed correspondingly. But her perception of the world had not changed in anything like the same degree. For it is our perception of the world that is important, not the mechanics of seeing. In a camera, optical quality may be paramount, but in the whole human apparatus of vision the desired end result is to gain a perception of the real world around us and decide whether we should be taking action. By the end of her seven days of experiment, she could cope with the world almost normally. The brain is able to make adaptations to accommodate changes in our senses; it learned in this case to cope with an inverted world and surprisingly did it very quickly. It must manage this trick by altering its processing of incoming information, information which is processed in only one way, by the firing of a chain of nerve cells. Whatever the mechanism by which vision is linked with the planning and execution of movements, that is quite different from the mechanism by which light enters the eye and is transformed into nerve signals. That process has been understood for some time, but it is now taking on a new significance in the light of the new theory of vision.

THE BRAIN IN THE EYE

The retina of the eye is already part of the brain. In our retinas there are millions of cells which are sensitive to light, and respond to various intensities, to changes in intensity, and to colours. Their responses are transformed into nerve signals, and travel from the retina via the optic nerve towards the back of the head and there enter the brain proper. From there the nerves lead to several different regions, which in some way turn the nerve signals into our perception of the visible world. How they do it, we don't yet know, but later in the chapter we shall see that there are theories which begin to explain this mysterious process. First let us look at some elements of the process, by investigating simpler eyes than ours.

The horseshoe crab, Limulus, is a living fossil, and it inhabits the Eastern shores of all the great oceans of the world. It grows to eighteen inches in diameter, looks rather like a frying pan with a domed lid and tapering pointed handle (the tail), and weights several pounds. It also has three pairs of eyes, which Dr Floyd Ratliff at Rockefeller University, New York, is studying to see what they can tell us about human vision.

Ratliff's laboratory developed a technique of connecting the optic nerve from one of the crab's eyes to an electrode, which recorded the responses of the nerve, and therefore of the eye, to light. One might expect the cells of the eye to produce a signal directly in relation to the intensity of light falling upon them, like the photo-electric cell in a light meter. Sure enough when a thin pencil beam of light was shone on to the eye, the optic nerve fired, but rather feebly. Dr Ratliff switched on the room lights too, to increase the firing, but instead the signal became even fainter. This seemed ridiculous, but several careful experiments established that it was entirely logical. The eye was not built to detect high or low light levels, but to respond to *changes* in light level across its surface. When the pencil beam of light was surrounded by darkness, the cells fired in response to the light/dark difference. When the room lights were switched on that difference was much less, so the cells responded less vigorously. This appreciation of changes in light intensity – not just the intensity itself – is a key feature of nature's process of visual perception.

Dr Ratliff relates this aspect of the primitive vision of the horseshoe crab to a human perception exemplified in a particular kind of Japanese painting, the sort in which the moon seems to stand out luminously in a comparatively dark sky. Cover all but two sections of such a painting – the moon and a part of the sky – with black paper, and it becomes obvious that both areas are in fact of the same light intensity. The apparent luminosity of the moon was produced by a contrast technique. The artist outlined the moon with a hard black line, then gradually reduced the blackness as he moved away into the sky, getting gradually to dark grey, then light grey, then white once again. The sharp white/black transition at the edge of the moon makes the white there seem whiter than the gradual light-grey/white transition into the sky. It is similar to the response of the crab to sharp boundaries between light and dark. There are optical illusions which produce the same effect. And when an artist uses his charcoal to draw the preliminary sketch for a painting, he is, at one level, outlining the shape of an object; but at another level he is merely indicating where light intensity changes

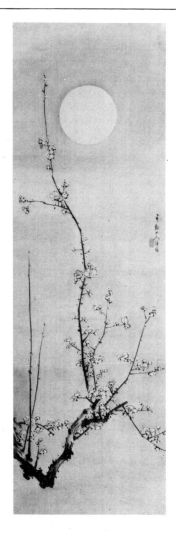
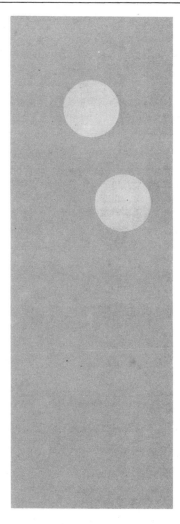

THE ILLUSORY MOON

The moon on the left appears to be brighter than the light part of the surrounding sky, but the mask on the right over the same picture shows that it is an illusion. Moon and sky are the same, and it is just one deft brush stroke by the artist which creates the effect. The eye is built to respond to changes in light intensity such as the sharp boundary round the moon and so assumes that the object itself is very light. Such inbuilt tendencies enable us to pick out objects in the real world.

abruptly. Changes in light level do tend to correspond with the outlines of objects: so we and Limulus have evolved to detect them.

In addition to the functional value of this initial step in the process of seeing, it serves the helpful purpose of reducing the amount of information that reaches the brain. Much information unnecessary to the operation of the 'seeing machine' in the brain does not even get passed along the optic nerve. If this were not the case, even the human brain could be overwhelmed with data.

INFORMATION FROM THE RETINA

Thus light signals have already been processed in the eye before they proceed, now as nerve impulses, along the optic nerves to the brain. With the information on light intensity goes the retina's response to colour and, possibly, movement. Nerve signals from the eyes go to both sides of the brain but there is a cross-over.

Information from the left visual field of each eye crosses to the right side of the brain and signals from the right visual field of each eye cross to the left side of the brain. These bundles of nerves run from the eyes under the brain, first past the surface of the thalamus to the lateral geniculate nucleus. The lateral geniculate nucleus seems to have a number of functions, but one appears to be further to sharpen contrast for processing in other regions of the brain. This interchange station is about half-way on the journey of the nerve signals from the eye to the visual cortex, at the back of the head. New nerve fibres come from the lateral geniculate nucleus, and make their way to a region low down at the back of the brain, called the visual cortex, or, because of its striped appearance under the microscope, the striate cortex. From the visual cortex, nerve messages are sent up and forward into the brain, to neighbouring regions in the cortex, and to other targets further down in the mass of the brain. The visual cortex is one of the best understood parts of the brain, because of experiments during the last twenty years.

BRAIN CELLS, AND SPECIFIC PERCEPTIONS

In 1981, David H. Hubel and Torsten N. Wiesel of the Harvard University Medical School were awarded the Nobel Prize for Medicine in recognition of their examination of the visual cortex of the cat. These studies began in 1959 and continued for several years, in the course of which Hubel and Wiesel mapped to an astonishing degree the organization of this part of the brain.

Hubel and Wiesel worked with an anaesthetized cat, whose open eye was directed at a screen on which different shapes were displayed. Vanishingly thin glass tubes were gradually inserted into the visual cortex. Their tips were narrow enough to puncture a single cell. Inside each of these micro-electrodes was a liquid which conducted the electrical signals of the punctured but still living cell to the recording apparatus. The results were quite astonishing. When the cat was shown a horizontal bar of light, for example, the electrode revealed that each cell in a column vertical to the surface of the cortex reacted similarly to the horizontal bar, but that a next-door column of cells would react best to a bar at a slightly different orientation, ten or fifteen degrees from the horizontal perhaps, and the next to a bar turned ten or fifteen degrees further, and so forth. There was not a sharp cut-off between the cells; cells on either side of the 'horizontal' reacting cells would still react to a horizontal stimulus, but it was possible to identify different columns responding best to different orientations of the bar. Moreover, groups of these columns were preferentially driven by either the right or the left eye, and these groups too were regularly arranged. It was possible to see these columns by stimulating the brain appropriately and then staining sections of it to reveal regions which have been recently most active. Hubel and Wiesel went on to

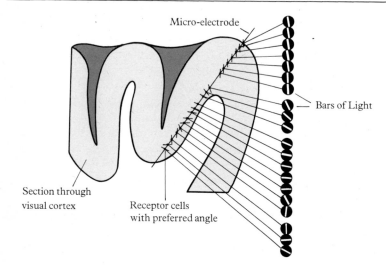

Micro-electrode

Bars of Light

Section through
visual cortex

Receptor cells
with preferred angle

ANGLES OF SEEING
The fields of the visual cortex in a
cat's brain are shown here cut
through and magnified. In their
pioneering work on vision David
Hubel and Torsten Wiesel inserted
a micro-electrode into the brain
and measured the firing of the cells
at various levels when the animal
was shown a moving bar of light at
various angles. Each cell
responded best to a bar at a
particular angle, shown on the
right. Presumably the cells'
response to such angles of lines in
the cat's field of view could be the
first stage in analysis of what is
being seen.

discover that, in addition to these 'bar orientation' cells, there were
other cells which responded to different particular features, such as
corners, and other more complex shapes.

If there are cells which respond to such specific stimuli as bars
at different angles, or corners, does this presuppose that there will
also be cells which respond to even more detailed features, to faces
perhaps, or even to particular faces? Do we have cells that recognize
our grandmothers? Is that what recognizing one's grandmother
actually and only involves? David Hubel says that this seems to him
to be unlikely, but that he has no good alternative to offer. We shall
see later in the chapter that an alternative interpretation has now
been developed. But as far as it shows how the brain itself is
organized in relation to its functions, the work of Hubel and Wiesel
is a giant step forward.

The discovery of the activity of specific small areas of the
brain and their relationship to particular kinds of pattern or shape
was thought, a decade ago, to promise enormous and rapid advance
in our understanding of the process of vision. Unfortunately, work
aimed at understanding further brain operations of the visual
system has not proceeded as fast as had been hoped. It is now clear,
too, that an individual cell in the visual cortex does not actually
detect a line of a particular orientation: its response is just not
specific enough. So we are still puzzling over the riddle of how the
brain is able to translate signals from the retina into a perception of
the real world.

When Susannah, with her inverted vision, really tried to do
active things she was able to manage quite remarkably difficult
tasks, like bicycling or cooking. She was learning to match her
vision with the signals reported by the rest of her body, touch,
hearing and so forth. She was not just seeing, but sampling the
world as a whole with her senses, and organizing them so that they

told stories which could be sensibly related to each other. She saw with her whole body, the whole apparatus of her senses, as it were, and not just with her eyes. Other work going on at Oxford suggests that many parts of the brain otherwise thought of as being concerned with functions not related specifically to vision do in fact come into play during the process of seeing and do not respond to any other sense.

THE HYPOTHETICAL GRANDMOTHER CELL

In the Oxford University Department of Experimental Psychology, Dr Edmund Rolls works with rhesus monkeys. Like Hubel and Wiesel, he uses micro-electrodes to examine the responses of cells in the brain. But Rolls uses monkeys which are awake and in pretty full command of their faculties. Rolls has found cells in the hypothalamus (the tiny part of the lower brain which deals with, among other things, regulation of body temperature, hunger and thirst) which respond to the sight of food. He is sure that he has eliminated any other possibility, and is left with the conclusion that these cells are for some reason specialized to respond to a visual signal about food. The cells are not specifically related to characteristic food objects, such as bananas; though they do fire at the sight of a banana. But they also fire at the sight of a black syringe, used to feed the monkey glucose, and not to fire when shown a white syringe which was used to give the monkey an unpleasant mixture of salt and water. They respond, therefore, to food associations, not to specific food shapes.

Perhaps the most surprising of all Rolls's results was the discovery of cells in a side portion of the brain, the superior temporal sulcus, which responded only to faces. Rolls tested fifty such nerve cells in two rhesus monkeys and discovered that all fifty of the cells responded to faces, either human or rhesus monkey, in three dimensions or projected in the flat, and did not respond to gratings or other simple or complex flat or three-dimensional objects. Further, some cells seemed to respond more strongly to features, like eyes or hair or the mouth. The faces in profile failed to get a response from some cells, but rotating or altering the colour or size of the full face did not much alter the response of the cells. Rolls believes that these cells may have developed the special function of responding to the sight of a face, perhaps since monkeys order their social grouping in hierarchies, and it may be important that monkeys do therefore recognize each other to obey the hierarchical rules of their society. But these cells may not be representative of the vast majority of nerve cells involved in the process of vision. Rolls has also found face-responding cells in parts of the amygdala, to which some fibres of the superior temporal sulcus run. There is some evidence, from studies in humans, that when similar pathways are interrupted it brings about a condition in which the patient is unable to recognize faces even of close relatives. So it is possible that the human brain also has cells specialized to help us recognize faces or facial features. Two notes of caution must be added, though. Firstly, Dr Rolls's research is controversial and has not yet been repeated by another researcher. Also, as Rolls himself admits, he may be looking at a rather unusual aspect of vision which is not typical of the seeing system.

It may be that the nerve cells Rolls associates with facial recognition do not respond only to visual input, and indeed, in view of the complex inter-connections of these areas of the brain, that seems likely. But the evidence does suggest that many other parts of the brain than we have hitherto thought possible may be connected with visual processing.

Work like that of Edmund Rolls is fascinating in itself, but brings to light profound differences in scientific approach. If we take into account Rolls's discovery of apparent face-recognition cells, and combine it with work like Hubel and Wiesel's discovery of bar orientation cells, together they tend to suggest that the brain works in a particular way: thus it may have a hierarchy of cells, with a large number of un-specialized cells feeding a small number of specialized cells. The simple cells will respond to and further refine gross aspects of the visual scene, and processing from that stage will reach on upwards until the most complex cells may respond to very specific visual stimuli: the grandmother cell will then respond only to grandmother's face.

It does seem to be true that in some areas the nervous system is arranged on various levels in this way. The motor system, for example, seems to have command cells, or groups of cells, which organize pre-programmed movements; and there are regions of the brain, very large groups of cells, which dominate the faculty of language (see Chapters 2 and 4 on language and movement). These are all hypotheses, though based on anatomical and physiological evidence. But the same evidence might fit a different hypothesis. The observation that the sun travels across the sky from east to west, for example, made Ptolemy believe that the sun was circumnavigating the earth, but the less obvious conclusion from this evidence, that the earth rotates on its axis, turned out to be the correct one. Ptolemy's system worked pretty well, in a practical way, and sailors were able to navigate by using it, even though it was absolutely incorrect. In the same way, one can form a theory of the functioning of the brain which would make rather good sense, using the principle of hierarchies. But in the last few years a theory has been developed which runs completely counter to this.

THE COMPUTATIONAL THEORY

Since digital computers became available, many scientists have found that it is valuable to compare the brain to a computer, and to use computers to simulate brain functions. There are probably more computers per square metre at the Massachusetts Institute of Technology than anywhere else in the world. Professor Whitman Richards works in the Artificial Intelligence Group at MIT, and he had this comment on the idea of the grandmother cells.

> If you have a sort of hierarchy, a collection of cells up there, grandmother cells or cells to react to every possible animal or thing that you might see, you're going to run out of cells very quickly. Think of all the possible objects, and size and shape or orientation that you could possibly encounter. You can put anything, a face for instance, in many different orientations and positions and distances and lighting conditions, and to each of those this single cell would have to respond. The brain's just going to run out of cells. It would require an infinite number, and an unlimited number of possible combinations between them. You cannot build a visual system out of grandmother cells.

Whitman Richards was a colleague and, he would probably agree, is a disciple of David Marr, a brilliant young Englishman who extended the horizons of many like Whitman Richards at MIT. We went to talk to David Marr, in the summer of 1980, in his rooms at Trinity College, Cambridge, where he was visiting. It was clear that he had one of the most original and creative minds ever to be brought to bear on the problems of brain function. After we saw him, Marr completed the major book on his own theory of vision on which he was working. He already knew that he had leukaemia and later in 1980, tragically, he died from it.

Although he had degrees in mathematics and in neurophysiology, Marr was latterly chiefly active in the theoretical studies which needed computers so badly. He told us that he had been obliged to leave Britain and go to MIT purely because nowhere else offered such computer power. But he was by no means a dry mathematical theorist. He began by thinking about what vision needed to do, namely to tell an animal about the physical world. Then he worked out what he thought would be the individual steps towards that achievement and expressed them in very precise form, as they must be in the brain, but also as they must be for simulation by computer. Then, because a theory must be tested, he began to build a vision machine at MIT incorporating his ideas. The machine has not yet been completed, but the process is still being carried on by his colleagues. Although David Marr expressed key concepts in his theory of vision in mathematical terms, it is beyond this book (or its authors) to explain these terms as they properly should be explained. But Marr could also address himself to innumerate listeners, and explain himself in terms which the layman could understand. Reasonably enough, Marr made use of references to the visual arts in his explanations, and in the simplified account which follows we shall take a cue from that to return to the painter whom we met earlier, Anthony Green. In many ways his starting point is also David Marr's starting point.

Anthony Green studied at the Slade School of Art, and there he was taught a particular technique. He was told how to look at things, and how to see what he was looking at. He was told that he should not have preconceived ideas but represent through his drawing the particular object which was his model. He did well, and when he left he won the Tonks Prize as the best draughtsman in the year. Just as that was his early approach, so it is the early approach of the visual system as interpreted by David Marr.

The eye and brain first process visual information about objects as presented to them, just as Anthony Green was taught to do at the Slade. The initial perception of the brain depends upon the person's point of view: a circular plate seen from an angle will actually be oval; and also, at this early stage of the seeing process, a face with bands of sunlight and shade slanting across it from a venetian blind will indeed be a face shape with some visible features and alternate light and dark bars across it. It will *not* be a *face* with a venetian blind pattern on it. A cow or deer will be a certain pattern of shape and colour and texture but not yet a cow or a deer. Already to reach this point the brain has done more than all the computers at MIT could do, but in order to achieve more precise visual perception of, say, an animal some more essential features must be extracted from the image.

Anthony Green seems now to have moved away from his early training in accurate representation and now he is often representing the artistic equivalent of generalized memory, the form in which we store and therefore recognize things. Green says:

> I think the view that I paint from is conditioned by my understanding of the personality of an object. Legs are leggy. Forks are forky. Newspapers are newspapery. I think we file them under what I call the personality of that object. Take the fork, for instance. It's no good painting a picture of a fork it looks as if it's made of india-rubber. A fork is a hard thing. It's got three or four prongs on it. It's forky. And this applies to ears, noses, mouths, whiskers, doors, whatever you want. They have a distinct personality which is understandable both to me and to everybody else. I think the personality is related probably to the function of the object: whether it stands four-square on the ground, whether it's hard or soft, whether you use it, whether it's mechanical, non-mechanical, soft, hard, whether you sit on it or eat it.

SEEING DOUBLE

In his painting, *Slave Market with the Disappearing Bust of Voltaire* (1940), Salvador Dali has created an illusion which the brain perceives either as the face of the philosopher Voltaire or three figures on a light background. When machines built to mimic the eye and brain respond to such illusions as well, we will have understood how human beings see.

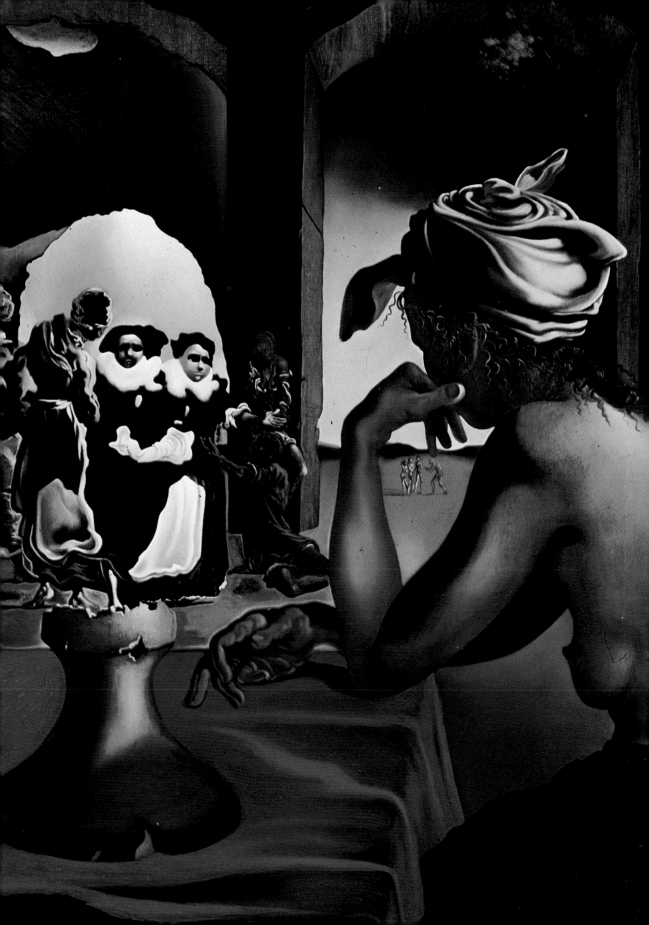

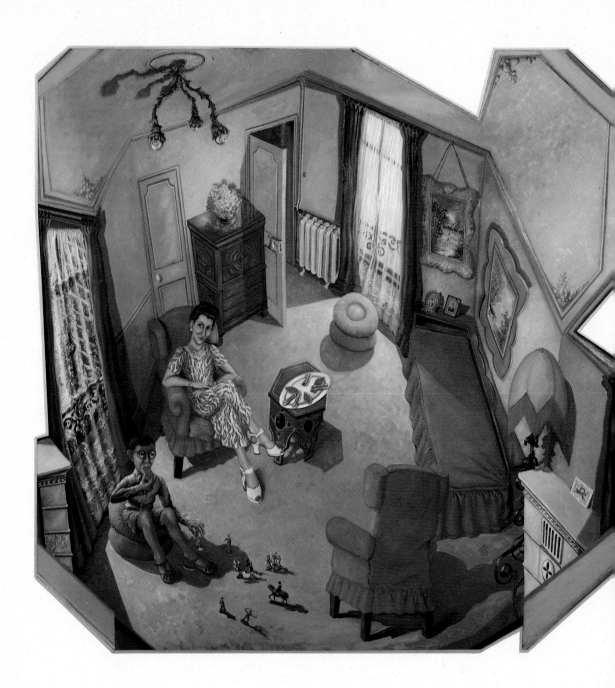

PICTURES FROM THE PAST
(*Left*) Anthony Green's painting, *Madame Madeleine Green et son fils. Raincy S et O. 1948* (1981). This artist's perception of doors, chairs, or a room from a range of apparently strange perspectives, may well mirror the images represented in the nerve cells of the brain.

(*Right*) Anthony Green, seen here in his studio, where he paints from images in his head and not from life.

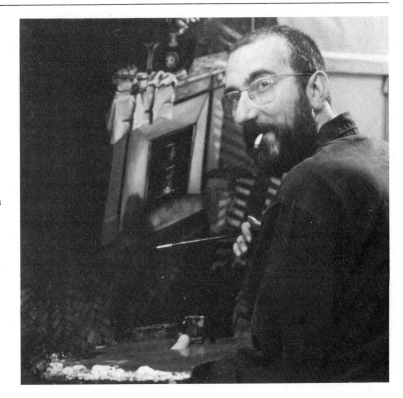

When he paints something Anthony Green is giving a generalized description of that particular object. From that description we are able to recognize the object. Humans (and perhaps monkeys) can go further and recognize particular objects, grandmothers' faces, for example. But we store what is basically a general description – *a* chair or *a* door, rather than that particular chair or that particular door. And the description is related to the object's function in our world. David Marr also believed that this is the way objects are recognized and stored in the brain.

Both men also realize that there is another essential for object recognition, which takes us back to the old idea of a cell in the brain which recognizes one's grandmother. One cell would not be enough. How many different lights, colours, or positions might she be found in? Each must have a cell. What happens when she smiles, frowns, opens her mouth, wears a veil? Each changes her face so much that to be able still to say, 'Hello, grandmother,' rather than, 'Hello, Mrs Green,' requires numerous cells for her alone, let alone for all the other relatives, people, animals, objects, and landscapes that we can all recognize. That cannot be the way the system works. First of all it must get rid of all the possible alternative aspects of an object by considering it from a fixed view-point. Then, somehow, the brain must convert the two-dimensional view projected onto the retina into a three-dimensional generalized structure rather than the eye's subjective view of it.

Anthony Green applies this principle to his recent paintings. He has begun to play with perspective, for instance, and to paint objects which are seen from more than one viewpoint at the same time.

> The pictures in my head are not from a fixed viewpoint. I simply know them. It's got nothing to do with art whatsoever. It's a knowing process. . . . When I come to make those visual memories tangible I have to go away from the concept of the professional artist who paints from a fixed viewpoint. Because how do you make those visual memories reality when you don't see them from a fixed viewpoint?

The effect of Anthony's theories about painting is sometimes curious, but it is always convincing. He seems to have the ability to extract the visual system's representations of the world from inside his head. Or at least, he extracts David Marr's version of the visual representation of the world.

David Marr believed that any visual process must be seen as proceeding to the end-point of providing an animal with a description of the world it sees. He looked for a way to extract from the viewed scene its implicit meaning – what Anthony Green might call 'forkiness'. At this end-point in the process of seeing, or

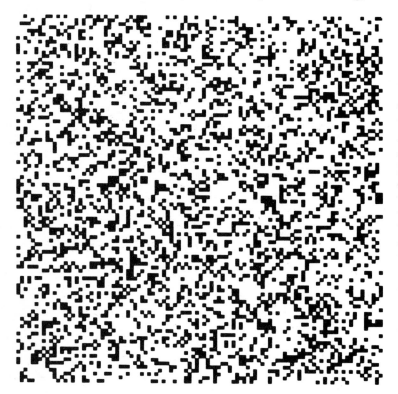

Left

STEREOSCOPIC VISION
These two patterns are random and each one contains no regular shape, but once they are combined in the brain, they make up a three-dimensional wedding cake shape. The shape only appears because the brain computes the similarities and differences between the dots in each image: a stupendous task. David Marr and his group worked out how it was done and to prove they were right built a machine to do the same thing.

To see the wedding cake: cut out each image. Place them on a table top a few inches apart and look down on them from a foot or more away. Hold a small mirror with its silvered side on the left side of your nose, so that your left eye views the mirror reflection on the left pattern and your right eye sees the right pattern directly. Move the patterns, head and mirror until perception, the brain should be able to sort through a catalogue of remembrances of things past and identify the object, either generally as a person, or particularly as a grandmother. That was the end-point to which the Marr theory had to lead.

A First Sketch

Marr was convinced that the brain's visual system could not be built on the basis of grandmother-recognizing cells because the computational problems would be too enormous. And, one suspects, he had an intuitive feeling that brains simply don't work that way. An interesting hint of the direction his detailed research might take came when he saw the so-called random dot stereograms devised by Bela Julesz at the Bell Laboratories in 1959. They consist of two apparently similar arrangements of numerous dots. These patterns appear to be without form when each is viewed by both eyes. But if matters are so arranged that the left can be viewed by the left eye alone and the right by the right eye alone, some of the dots outline a recognizable simple shape, such as a square. So the brain was recognizing features in images that *had* no features. Where did this leave the grandmother cell, or any of the theory based on it?

Marr became more convinced that the feature-detecting cell idea would not wash. He began to look for a process that would

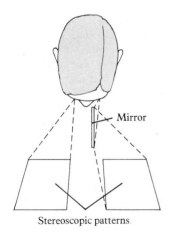

Mirror

Stereoscopic patterns

the two images coincide. It may take a few minutes as your brain is having to carry out billions of computations. Do not strain. The effect, once achieved, is striking.

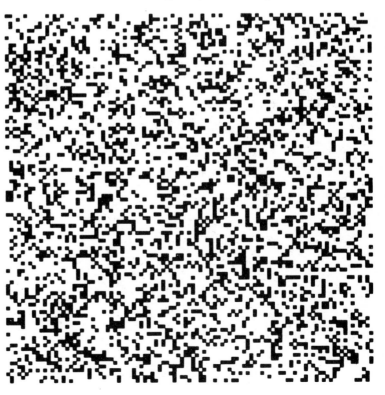

Right

make an object recognizable at a very coarse level and with the minimum of information. The random dot stereogram gave the obvious answer: Julesz had constructed the stereogram by making a proportion of the dots different in the pattern presented to each eye. The brain, reasoned Marr, must therefore be comparing the pattern of dots from one eye with the pattern from the other, working out which ones were different and concluding that the differences outlined a square. But to take all the dots from the left eye and compare them with all the dots' positions in the right eye is a computational task of gigantic proportions. Obviously there must be a series of approximations carried out by the brain (unconsciously because we never experience them) which gets progressively finer until eventually the brain homes in on the few dots, among many thousands, that are actually different in each eye. But on what form of brain input was the computation done? It was, Marr discovered, done on the intensity change representation coming down the optic nerve to the striate cortex. This was in the form of a rough sketch of the changes from light to dark all over each eye's image. 'Sketch' is the right word in the sense that it was an outline of the major features, much like an artist's rough charcoal sketch, but of course it was *not* a picture but a series of signals about light/dark transitions expressed as nerve cells firing or not firing. Also, it could somehow be 'looked at' mathematically by the brain at various resolutions, rather as if it was at first examined out of focus;

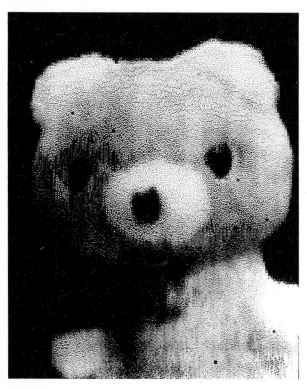

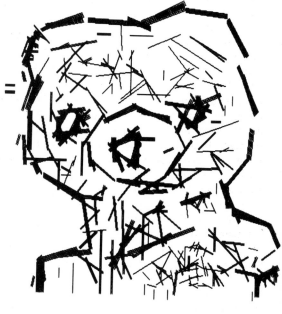

then the brain gradually homed in on the important parts by 'focusing' more and more all the time. This so-called 'primal sketch' was, Marr believed, the first crucial stage of all vision. Intuitively, it seems convincing. A skilled artist, such as David Hockney, can convey a surprising amount by a few black lines which are actually following the main changes in intensity. They are the places where the brain cells fire fastest when we look at the real object rather than the drawing. The sketch can tell us not only what is being depicted, but identity and character.

Marr reasoned that the 'primal sketch' used the contrast-detecting cells which he knew to be present in such creatures as the horseshoe crab and are also present in our own eyes. Simple cells like these would be able to determine boundaries of light and shade and therefore sketch in the shape of an object, albeit a fairly crude representation.

BUILDING A VISION MACHINE

Theories are all very well, but Marr was anxious to see if his theory worked. So he built a vision machine based on a computer. He and his colleagues devised mathematical processes which would fulfil the various assumptions that the theory made. The computer was programmed to produce primal sketches of objects from the electrical output of a television camera. Given its instructions, the computer produced its primal sketch, a crude but recognizable facsimile of a teddy bear's head. It had been detected by computer equivalents of the eye and brain and although the program allowed it to be viewed, to check its accuracy, it was in the form of stored electrical signals, not a picture.

Next, stereopsis. Again, it was possible for Marr and his colleagues to work out a mathematical method of computation which, this time, enabled the computer to 'see' the concealed pattern in a random dot stereogram using the 'primal sketch'. Next, one of Marr's collaborators, Shimon Ullman, devised a mathematical technique for computing the structure of an object from its motion. Just as stereopsis involved comparing the primal sketch from each eye's slightly different dot patterns, so detecting movement was a comparison of the input at one point in time with that an instant later. Imagine a spotted dalmatian dog against a similarly spotted background. When the dog is stationary, it cannot be seen: there are not enough visual cues to distinguish the dog. (It is camouflaged, and of course many animals use just this technique in the wild.) The instant the dog moves, the brain decides what it is; this must be interpreted from movement alone. To recognize the animal the brain first has to decide from one moment to the next which spots are the same but have moved, and which are actually different spots. If the wrong spots were chosen, the result would be a visual error, what we call an illusion. Shimon Ullman carried out

DAVID MARR'S BEAR
This trivial object could go down in history as the most significant contribution to our understanding of the brain. David Marr developed a theory which precisely defined what the brain needed to do in order to see. He and his collaborators built a machine to mimic the very first steps of seeing and its first effort was the image on the right. In the machine, as in the brain, there is of course no actual image, but a pattern of electrical signals which for clarity are here converted back into a visual image. The machine has succeeded in extracting and simplifying the information from the bear which outlines its important features. The final stage will be to build a machine which will actually recognize an object.

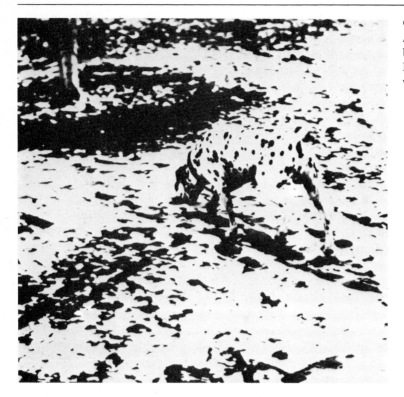

CAMOUFLAGE
An apparently random set of blotches, which camouflage a Dalmatian. If the dog moved, it would be instantly recognizable.

further tests to check his technique, and in doing so discovered that the brain stores a variety of assumed knowledge about visual images. One very basic assumption in the case under study was that an image which is a very precise representation of a dog is reckoned by the brain to be an image of a single object (although it is quite possible to put together a collection of objects to assume the shape of a single dog). Another, related to an object in motion, is that the brain assumes that a moving image on the retina comes from a three-dimensional object. But the brain can be deceived in this instance, too. The MIT computers can construct, by displays of moving dots, objects which the brain judges to be three-dimensional. Of course, they are not, but when the computer-made 'objects' move in a manner consistent with their real-life equivalents, the visual system is always fooled.

It seems, therefore, that we are far more at the mercy of the assumptions built into our brains than we would ever have supposed. Marr and Ullman make their own assumption, that such processes are carried out by the brain in the course of constructing 'primal' sketches.

Many kinds of information can be derived from the primal sketch, just as Marr hoped. And the machine which has been built, incorporating the computer, is, so far, behaving like the human visual system. Perhaps the most convincing evidence of this is that it is fooled, just as we are, by optical illusions. And, whatever we may

IMPOSSIBLE TRIANGLE
At first sight this seems to be a complete 3D triangle, but the details make it clear that it is an impossible object and two sides do not join. Once a vision machine is built, illusions like this can be used to test whether it works like the human eye and brain. If the machine is fooled at first, it must work on similar principles to the brain.

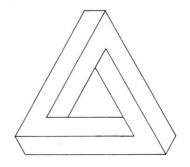

not know about computers, we know that they don't have pictures in their heads. All they have is a memory composed of information coded in binary form, just on or off.

THE ANALOGY OF THE WEATHER MAP

But if the computer, or our nerve cells for that matter, aren't drawing a picture in our heads, what are they doing? If Marr is right, it is some form of computation. The mathematics are distinctly formidable, but one can use the analogy of the familiar weather map to understand the sort of computation that takes place.

On a weather map there are graceful curving lines showing low or high pressure areas. But there are no such lines in the North Sea. They are derived from many single observations at single points, just like the information taken in by the eyes. Those observations have to be collected, processed to extract from them the essential mathematical summary of the weather, just as the brain does with visual information. Then the weather map is drawn. Various features are already evident: just as at this stage of vision the brain may be responding to an object's overall shape, so it may be evident that the weather is bad. The equivalent to 'seeing' is actually using the weather map to decide what to do: whether to risk a boat trip or a flight or even a walk outside. Like weather forecasting, seeing is there only to enable us to make informed decisions about the world. When the weather is monitored and compared from one hour to the next, this information can be used to predict with at least a little certainty what will happen next, just as we can discern in which direction an animal may be moving by continuously sampling various items of information in our visual system. While weather is broken down into temperature, pressure and humidity, Marr broke down the analysis of a visual scene by the brain into movement, stereopsis, colour, texture, and so forth. At the later, post-primal-sketch stages of seeing, the brain finally begins to implement Anthony Green's thinking and recognize objects as themselves.

Marr believed that the brain recognizes objects by using several elements. One he called the stick figure model: all the brain has to compute to recognize such a figure as rabbit, giraffe, ostrich or goat is the length and angle of each stick. At the next stage, the brain specifies the relative size of the trunk, limbs, and antlers by 'drawing' cylinders round these axes. Of course our visual impression of a deer is much richer than this: we use colour, texture and so on, but Marr had not found a solution to this aspect of the problem before his untimely death. All these processes are going on, not one after another, but simultaneously and at enormous speed, and at the end-point are compared by the brain with a 'catalogue' of known objects – in short, recognized. So far, only the computations for the primal sketch stage have been devised and built into the

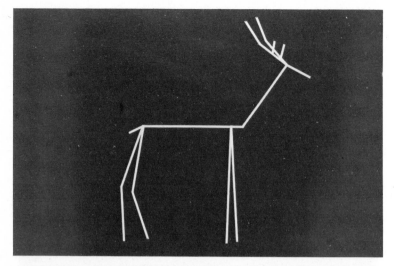

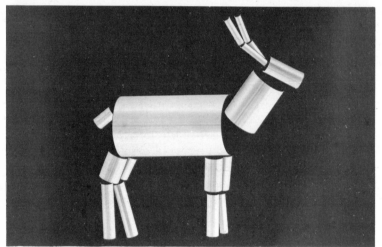

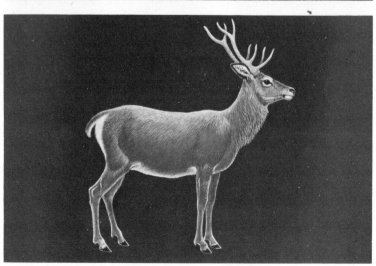

REPRESENTATION IN THE BRAIN

The stick figure on the left contains very little information compared to the full deer at the bottom, yet we are able to recognize it. David Marr proposed that the brain's nerve cells may be organized to construct a non-visual version of a stick figure when we look at an object, especially an animal, and it is stored in our memories, to be compared with our next view of an animal. The deer's bulk may be simply represented as cylinders round the axes of the stick figure. Once these are joined in the brain by visual information on colour, texture and so on, we perceive a deer in its full detail.

vision machine at MIT. The last stage, of comparing incoming information with the catalogue, will certainly stretch any existing computers to their limits, or beyond them.

IMPRESSIONISM

If the assumption that the brain can derive enough information to recognize objects or people from what appear to be very simple elements seems hard to swallow, we may perhaps turn again to painting to illustrate the point and, we hope, convince the reader. The example of the black and white drawing has already been given. But we can almost certainly derive as much information from pure colour. Impressionist paintings of the nineteenth century, Monet's water lilies for example, are composed of flat planes of colour; but when we see the pictures we get an instant impression of a scene in three dimensions in which we can 'recognize' many details that are not really there. The painter has not painted the details. We derive them from our fleeting impression of the scene. And one can sense from such paintings not only shape and form and colour, but even the direction of light and the warmth of the sun.

The artist Anthony Green has a perfect understanding of the process. 'I'm not a camera,' he says, 'I'm a seeing and remembering machine with a soul, and that complicates the issue terribly.'

The issue – how do we see the world – is certainly a complicated one. But each step we have discussed has taken our knowledge towards understanding. We can describe in detail what the nervous system does: the processing of vision by the retina, the relaying of that information by the lateral geniculate nucleus, the columns of cells in the visual cortex, and the branching pathways that run to so many other parts of the brain. But we cannot look at even these complex details in isolation from the allied processes in which the brain is involved: memory, movement, hunger or emotion. Uncannily, an artist can tap into all these sources in a way which the camera cannot. David Marr's theory may be only the beginning of an understanding of the brain, and it may be overturned tomorrow. But it does seem to be asking the right questions, and without the right questions we shall never get the right answers.

Seeing is a function over which we have no physical influence. When we open our eyes, if we *can* see then we will. In the next chapter, which deals with movement, we arrive at a faculty which, while in some ways physically simpler, involves the intentions and the will.

CHAPTER 4

MOVEMENT

The previous chapter dealt with a form of brain input, vision, and we now discuss a fundamental form of output, movement. The two are linked in the nervous system by processes which vary from the simplest to, arguably, the most complex we perform. We shall pay appropriate attention to the structures of the brain and the functions those structures perform, and we shall examine the role of the spinal cord in movement. This analysis will take us closer yet to mechanisms, but above all to understanding what we mean by a machine, and whether we can agree and accept that the human being is a machine or not.

A MATTER OF LIFE OR DEATH

The difference between a dead thing and a live thing is movement, and under the terms of that definition human beings are different from stones. But are they different from machines? Machines are often in restless movement, wheels spinning, levers thrashing, pistons pumping. Within the circuits of a computer, though we can no more see them than we can see the back of the moon, electric charges are in constant movement. Is it not possible to believe that man is an almost perfect machine for movement?

Indeed, if we pause to think for a moment about our own movements, we must acknowledge that many of them are automatic, or machine-like. Our hearts beat, and we breathe, and our intestines contract without our giving any thought to the matter. Even at a higher level, we still do not have to think about most of our movements. We pick up a pen or put it down without consciously considering the action, and if we are hurrying for a bus, we give no thought to the actions of our legs; we do not direct the left and then the right to move alternately, nor do we command our heels to hit the ground before our toes. All those things happen automatically, and it is with the current research into these automatic processes that we begin our investigation of the brain's involvement in movement.

CAN BABIES WALK?

The Karolinska Institute in Stockholm is one of the world's most powerful research organizations, and one of the Institute's interests is the nervous control of walking and running. The Institute's director is Professor Sten Grillner, one of the most respected scientists in the field of movement.

In the Physiology Institute, Grillner has a huge treadmill, about 25 feet long, on which his experimental subjects walk. He also has a much smaller model, turned by hand, on which, amazingly, babies walk. And they really are babies, of between four and six weeks. The infant is comforted and supported, raised to a standing position and placed on the treadmill which one of the assistants starts to turn. In most instances the baby starts to walk. It is clear that this is not merely a case of legs moving under the influence of the moving treadmill. It is a real walk, one leg after the other, and the foot rolling to contact the ground. But babies can't walk. How can this be explained?

At this early age, it seems, the baby still possesses and can use the inbuilt walking mechanism with which it was endowed by its genes. The nerve cells controlling the mechanism, probably in the spine, are not yet under the full control of the brain, and the baby's nervous system is, as it were, at an early stage of evolution. One of Grillner's colleagues, Dr Forssberg, has examined the phenomenon of the walking baby in some detail. He believes that the baby-walk is like the walk of an animal such as the cat which moves about on four legs. The baby's foot hits the ground toes first, as do the feet of all animals, except man, during walking. It has been known for many years that a cat whose spinal cord has been severed below the brain, so that its movements are not under the control of the brain, can walk, and indeed run, quite successfully on a treadmill. Of course, one would not sever a baby's spinal cord in the same way, but it is

PATTERNS OF WALKING
A comparison of the angles of leg joints between the 'walking reflex' of a young baby and a child just beginning to walk. The pattern will continue to change until adolescence.

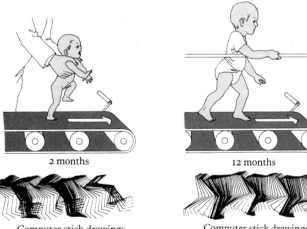

2 months   12 months

Computer stick drawings   Computer stick drawings

plain nevertheless that the baby's walking is not, at this age, under the control of its developing brain. At birth the nervous system is still not fully developed, and adult forms of walking may depend on nerve pathways only completed later in life.

The baby does not just happen to walk. What, then, is the control system which puts its limbs and joints into the appropriate positions at the appropriate time? Grillner believes that there are specialized cells in the spinal cord which generate patterns of nerve impulses to move the right muscles at the right time to produce the motions of walking. The baby will lose the walking movements from about six weeks old, and regain them in full only when it starts true walking, at 12 or 18 months. Then, says Grillner, it will also have the control of balance which a two-legged, upright-walking animal needs. Grillner and Forssberg have studied walking and running up to adulthood in man, and analysed the movements in great detail. To do this they attach infra-red 'lights' to the limbs, and photograph them with a special television camera, which also records its output onto a computer, which draws 'stick figures'. The resulting diagrams give them angles for joints at hip, knee, ankle and toe involved in walking and running, so that they can identify muscles which have to be used; and used differently, of course, for walking and for running.

PATTERN GENERATOR CELLS FOR MOVEMENT

It seems that there may be separate pattern generator cells for walking and running in man; there is evidence that they exist in cats and other animals. The brain, presumably, instantly switches from one pattern to another at the appropriate time as a run succeeds a walk, and the spinal cord pattern generator cells carry on the movement until it is countermanded by the brain. While it seems that all vertebrate animals have such pattern generator cells, their presence in man can only be inferred.

It may, therefore, not be quite accurate for us to speak of a child learning to walk. Parts of his walking mechanism may be almost as fully developed when he is born as the walking mechanism of the deer, which can stand up and run within minutes of birth. It may instead be that the brain has to learn how to control an inbuilt walking mechanism, and to maintain balance. It is a subtle but an important difference.

The presence of pattern generators for movements like walking give us the opportunity of moving without thinking. Our brains are spared the trouble of supervising all the stages of walking or running, and given more opportunity to pay attention to important problems, like finding bus-stops or avoiding lamp-posts. But the living human brain and spinal cord are too precious to dissect or damage to search for pattern generators; they are also too complicated.

LESSONS FROM THE LAMPREY'S SPINE

Locomotion, if not walking, can be studied at much higher resolution in the simpler nervous system of lower vertebrates, whose spinal cords are early sketches, as it were, for man's spinal cord. The animal which is Professor Grillner's choice is the lamprey. It is an unlovable creature, a fish lower in the evolutionary scale than ordinary fishes, without scales or jaws, but with a round mouth set with sharp teeth by which it attaches itself to its prey. Its only real attraction is a simple nervous system, which has relatively few nerve cells, that can be studied far more easily than the complex nerve networks of higher animals.

The lamprey swims rather like a snake moves. In each spinal segment its muscles are activated alternately, so that the body generates a wave which travels along with increasing amplitude, and pushes the creature forward through the water. Each spinal segment of the lamprey contains only three or four hundred nerve cells. To an expert physiologist it is a relatively simple matter to design experiments with it.

Just as cats do not need their brains for walking, so the lamprey does not need its brain for swimming. A so-called spinal lamprey, one in which the spinal cord has been severed below the brain, will begin its characteristic sinuous swimming movements when held facing upstream in flowing water. Clearly, while the movements could not be switched on or off or varied by the brain, the cord itself was able to generate them without the intercession of the brain.

It would be a mistake to think that, because the spinal cord has a built-in mechanism for swimming in lampreys, or for walking in land animals, that these forms of locomotion are entirely automatic. Clearly, the brain remains in command. As Professor Grillner says,

> The brain has one reasonably simple task, and that is to initiate the stereotyped movements that result in propulsion, and to decide whether those movements should be slow, fast, or very fast. Another more complex problem that the brain has is how to adapt these movements to the requirements of the animals, so that animals, including man, can reach the goals which they aim for. We know comparatively little about that type of control.

PROGRAMS

Professor Grillner calls such motor cells in the spinal cord 'pattern generators'. The procedures of swimming or walking which these pattern generator cells play out are usually referred to, in language derived from the computer, as programs. (This version of the spelling is the one adopted by computer scientists internationally.) The lamprey's swimming program, then, can be compared to the program stored in the memory of a computer which causes it to carry out certain functions; one could compare it to the program of an industrial robot. And, as in the case of a robot, the program may be replaced. In order to carry out its process (welding car bodies, painting furniture, or whatever) the robot must initially be provided with a set of instructions, on disc or tape. But if the process it is required to carry out needs to be changed, the instructions will need to be re-written, and a new program provided. Many robots can be re-programmed by taking them through each step of the required process once; after this the new program, which has been recorded during the rehearsal, as it were, comes into play. This distinction is also the distinction between innate programs and learned programs in animal movement. Some programs appear to be innate, to be born with the animal, like the baby's walking program which Grillner and Forssberg have investigated. But there must also be learned programs which will deal with requirements that have not been predicted by our genes. So most of us would regard changing gear in a car as a pretty automatic process, and indeed it can be described as a learned program: a fairly complex set of movements which is stored in our memories and translated into muscle action when necessary; but it was not born with us, like the program for walking. Our genes did not predict the motor-car, but they provided us with the flexibility to learn to use it.

If a robot has a program for carrying out spot-welding on a car body, as long as the car body arrives on the exact point on the line for which the robot is programmed, all will be well. But if the car body arrives a few inches away from its required position, the robot will make its welds in the wrong place, with disastrous results. Similarly, an animal may have a program for walking, but the program could not accommodate unexpected circumstances, such as a rock or a river which the animal must negotiate. The animal must react to unexpected circumstances, sometimes very quickly indeed, and there must therefore be a means of coming out of the program and taking action to deal with unpredicted situations.

CHANGING THE PROGRAM

We are equipped with organs receiving signals from our environment which help us to make such changes in our movements. We can, above all, *see* that circumstances have changed, if there happens to be a fallen tree or a broken paving-stone in our path. To a somewhat lesser degree, we may hear or feel changes in our environment which may signal an unexpected feature. But there is another sense upon which we depend, in particular in the case of movement. This is the sense of our own body in space – our sense of ourselves. This sense is largely derived

ROBOT PROGRAM
Industrial robots, like these at
work in a British Leyland factory,
can be programmed to move in an
exact sequence. In this respect
they move like an animal with a
spinal cord but no brain.

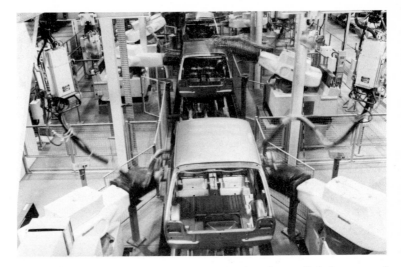

from sense organs in our muscles which tell us of their state of
tension. So our brains can register information not only about our
environment, but about our position in it and the arrangement of
our limbs, and use all this information to adapt the learned or
inbuilt programs which otherwise give the instructions which
enable us to walk or swim. And we need to be able to make very
rapid changes from one mode of operation, the programmed, to the
other mode of operation in which we react to circumstances: to
jump over the fallen tree.

This is particularly sophisticated in the case of skilled, learned
movements, such as those involved in playing a musical instrument.
A pianist's movement system may possess programs which give him
the skill to play the piano in the first place, and to play a particular
concerto in the second. These are learned programs. But he will
need also to react to the tempo chosen by the conductor, the skill of
the accompanying musicians, and the particular characteristics of
the instrument he is playing, stiff keys or pedals, for instance.
Therefore, while for the most part he is obeying the instructions of
his learned programs, stored in his nervous system, the same
nervous system is enabling him to react constantly to more or less
unexpected situations.

MOVEMENT, AND DISEASES OF THE NERVOUS SYSTEM

Dr Edward Evarts, at the United States National Institute of
Mental Health, began his scientific career in medical school, and
although he now devotes himself purely to research, the aim of his
work is clearly directed at an understanding of the various diseases
of movement associated with the nervous system, and their possible
prevention. Cure, he points out, is difficult to achieve in the human
nervous system, which exhibits only very limited capacity for
regenerating itself.

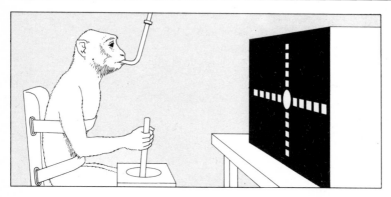

BERT'S GAME
Bert the monkey has to try to use his handle to keep the lamp in the centre of the cross alight, while his arm is randomly pushed or pulled. In this experiment, Bert has to 'change his mind' between voluntary and automatic modes of operation.

Evarts works with patients suffering from diseases like Parkinson's Disease or Huntington's Chorea. But because some forms of research involving the implantation of electrodes cannot be done with human subjects, he, like Professor Grillner, must also work with animals, chiefly with monkeys, whose nervous system as higher primates more closely resembles the nervous system of humans.

Because the brain operations in which Evarts is interested are extremely complex, a subject monkey must be taught tasks which involve the use of as many parts of his brain as possible; Bert is one of Evarts's best-behaved monkeys, who is undergoing a course of training in a game like a simplified form of 'Space Invaders'. The monkey is buckled into a chair in front of an array of lights in the shape of a cross. The centre of the cross is a tiny red light, and the arms of the cross consist of about eight segments of tiny green lights. Bert's task is to keep the red light in the centre of the cross alight as long as possible; and while he succeeds he gets supplied with orange juice from an automatic dispenser. No red light, no orange juice. But the job is not as easy as it looks, because the arm with which Bert operates the lever to keep the red light going is alternately pushed and pulled at random by an evil-minded computer nearby. So Bert has to change continually from the easy job of lighting the red light by pushing the lever in the appropriate direction to the more difficult one of overcoming the unpredictable push or pull on his arm. It is certainly not easy, but Bert is getting rather good at the game, and his orange juice keeps flowing.

When Bert has learnt his game, he will be taken to an operating theatre where a tiny electrode will be inserted into his brain and cemented to his skull. The electrode will be eavesdropping on the activity of particular brain cells, and Evarts will choose which brain cells it is that he needs to monitor, to establish how signals in the brain pass from one area to the other, in what order, and how long they take. To choose a target for the electrode, of course, he must know which part of the brain does what, at least as far as possible. Evarts explained to us which parts of the brain were known to be involved in movement. On the roof of the brain, the

A PURKINJE CELL
(*Opposite, above*) This is the most spectacular cell in the cerebellum. The maze of dendrites which receive messages can be seen clearly, and the axon can be faintly seen just below the cell body. The axons transmit the main signals from the cerebellum.

CIRCUITRY OF THE CEREBELLUM
One part of the cerebellum's surface, or cortex, is much like another (*see diagram opposite*). The black and yellow cells are inhibitory and interact with the blue excitatory cells to influence the output of the red Purkinje cells, through some 200,000 contacts on each cell.

(*Following colour page*)
CELLS CONNECTED WITH MOVEMENT
The cells in the motor cortex (*above left*) are involved in the regulation of movement. The Golgi stain used darkens only about one cell in a hundred, making it possible to see their fibres and relationships. In the low magnification 'slice' (*below left*), the band of dark-coloured cells shows up as a layer near the surface of the brain. The paler areas contain message-carrying fibres wrapped in fatty insulating sheaths.

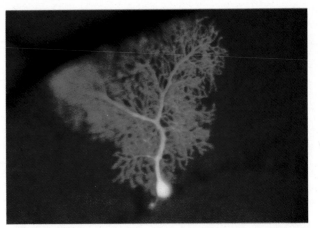

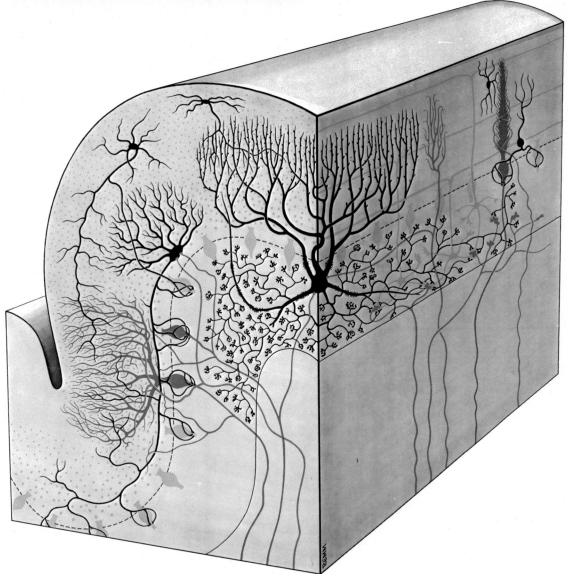

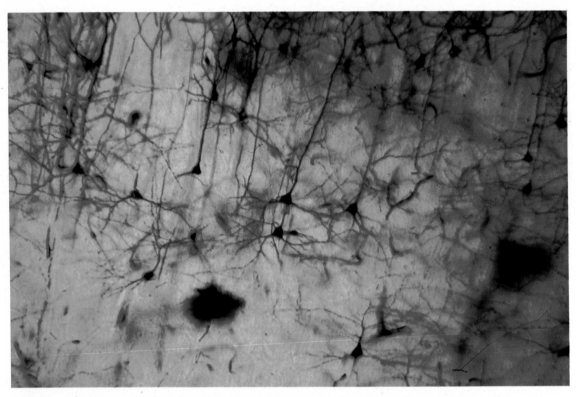
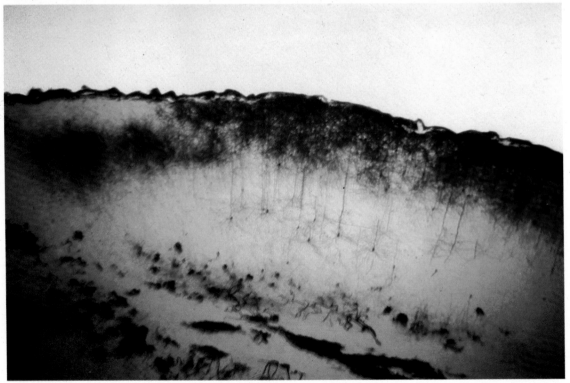

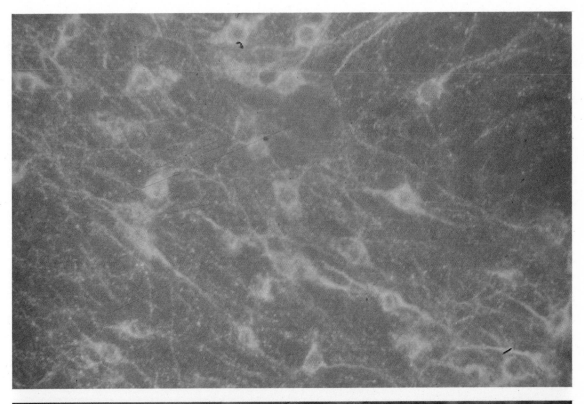

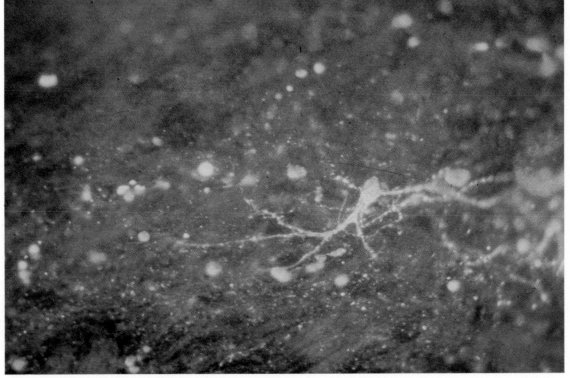

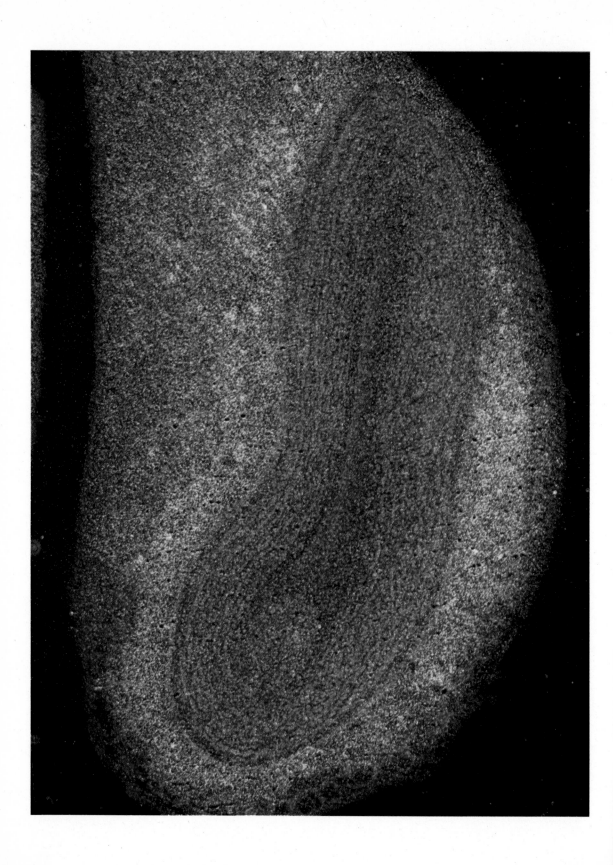

Fear and the Receptors of
Calm
(*Left*) Radioactive Valium shows
up the receptors in this section of
a rat's brain. The light yellow
area shows a concentration of
receptors which are thought to
play a part in the relief of anxiety
(*see page 140*).

(*Previous colour page*)
Tracing Parkinson's
Disease in the Brain
(*Above right*) These are cells in
the substantia nigra, stained to
glow green under ultra violet
light. It is the destruction of these
cells, by unknown causes, that is
responsible for Parkinson's
Disease (*see page 119*).

(*Previous colour page*)
(*Below right*) The pale yellow-
green cell just to the right of
centre is an embryo cell
transplanted into a rat's brain. The
fibres branching from it have
grown after transplantation (*see
page 121*).

cerebral cortex, there are three regions involved in voluntary
movements – like playing Space Invaders. At the front, under the
forehead, one area seems to set goals. It communicates with the
motor cortex, at the top of the head, which communicates with a
next-door area just behind the sensory strip of cortex to which our
sense-organs communicate. In very skilful, precise activities, like
playing the piano, feedback between sensory and motor cortex is
very important. Below the cortex, other regions are concerned with
movement. The cerebellum, a bulge at the back of the brain, sends
messages to the thalamus, almost at dead centre, which also
connects with the basal ganglia, just behind; and both the basal
ganglia and the cerebellum also send messages to the motor cortex
by way of the thalamus. After all these brain areas have done their
job, it is from the motor cortex that long nerve fibres run down to
the spinal cord where they operate motor nerve cells which send
instructions to the muscles.

The Order of Events in Movement

It is simply not possible to give an unequivocal account of the order
of events which initiate a voluntary or willed movement. Our
understanding of the brain may be approaching that level, but
before it can be attained even more accurate anatomical surveys
need to be made to plot the many millions of interlocking pathways
in the brain, and we have to tap into all of them before the order of
events can be precisely established. So can we describe the events in
the brain of the concert pianist, and relate them to movement?
Events in the brain take place so rapidly and so continuously that a

Tracing Movement in a
Monkey's Brain
(*Right*) The thick arrows
represent messages from various
parts of the cortex. Subsequent
reprocessed messages run from
the basal ganglia and the
cerebellum through the thalamus
to the motor cortex, which relays
them to the spinal cord.

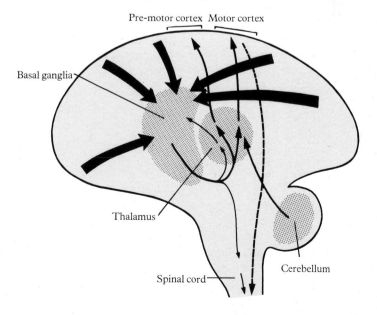

Pre-motor cortex Motor cortex

Basal ganglia

Thalamus

Spinal cord

Cerebellum

simplified sequence may be almost meaningless. But it may be helpful to give such a simplified sequence, with many reservations; and it may go something like this. The conductor raises his baton, and the pianist prepares to play. The baton descends. First the frontal area of the pianist's cortex, connected with goals and intentions, becomes active. This presumably makes a plan for the movement that is about to take place. The plan will then be processed in other cortical regions, and in the cerebellum and basal ganglia. At the next stage, the motor cortex will come into action, and relay its messages via the brain stem to the spinal cord. The pianist's fingers strike the piano keys. At the same time, the sensory cortex will be reporting back to other brain centres on the progress of the movement.

It is work like that of Dr Evarts which will ultimately give an accurate account of such events, and it should eventually be of interest not only to those concerned in pure research but for clinical purposes. If it is possible for us to understand the precise order of brain events, we will be able to identify the stage at which the brain makes an error in disorders of movement like Parkinson's Disease, with its disturbing tremor and stiffness of movement.

Already Evarts's work with monkeys has established that brain areas are active long before movement takes place; recordings from a motor cortex cell will rise to a peak substantially before the animal's muscles are activated. Clearly, the brain is in a constant ferment of action before the body moves. But we should be clear that this brain activity is not necessarily conscious activity. This leads us to re-examine critically the question of the brain's involvement in movements of an automatic or mechanical nature.

THE REFLEX

When Bert played his game, because the machine could randomly jog his arm, he might have to 'change his mind' about an intended move in order to fight the machine, light the red lamp, and get his orange juice. Evarts identifies the responses that require such precise control as being reflex: that is, regulated by signals back from the sense-receptors in Bert's arm. Just the same interplay takes place when the pianist plays, though his skill is so much more developed than Bert's; or when a marksman steadies his rifle to take aim at a target. However precise our movements, we are largely unconscious of the means by which we achieve them. So even voluntary and precise movements have a component which is reflex, or automatic. But what is a reflex?

To understand the concept of the reflex we need to look back some eighty or ninety years to the theories of the great pioneer investigator of nervous systems, Sir Charles Sherrington. Sherrington's theories have a permanent place in our conception of the nervous system, and they were based firmly on experiment. At least part of his success lay in his skill in caring for his experimental animals, which all too often in the later nineteenth century died at the hands of experimentalists; however critical his operations, Sherrington's animals usually survived them.

In the nineteenth century the sneeze and the cough were quoted as the examples, par excellence, of the reflex: if a hair tickled the nose, a sneeze was automatic – a reflex action. Similarly, a crumb in the throat would cause a cough automatically, another reflex action. The reflex with which most of us are familiar is the knee jerk, invariably used in neurological examinations to establish the health of nerve pathways to and from the spinal cord. But, as Ed Evarts says, the knee jerk is only a 'laboratory reflex'. It is not one which is used in our day-to-day activity, though it is undoubtedly a reflex. Even that, though, was in doubt in Sherrington's time because of ignorance of basic nerve anatomy.

In the course of his investigation of the knee jerk reflex Sherrington was obliged to make the most detailed anatomical and physiological experiments. Sherrington established that there is in the muscle a sensory nerve which informs the spinal cord of the state of stretch existing in the muscle. The tap on the tendon below the knee stretches the muscle. The stretch detector, through its nerve fibre, signals to a nerve in the spinal cord that the muscle is stretched, and that nerve then contracts the muscle to restore equilibrium. Two nerve cells are involved, and their action is pre-determined: once the stretch has taken place, the contraction will follow automatically. While the knee jerk in itself is not a 'real' reflex, since it serves no useful purpose except to neurologists, one can see how such a corrective mechanism would operate to our advantage, particularly in the matter of standing upright. If a muscle is detected to be stretching without our intending it, say on the deck of a rolling ship in a rough sea, the likelihood is that we will fall over unless compensatory action is taken. Thus, this simple variety of reflex helps us to maintain our upright posture.

Sherrington went further, and in a classic experiment established that a dog without a brain will still scratch when bitten by a flea. Sherrington operated to cut the spinal cord below the brain, and using what he described as an 'electric flea', which he rigged up from an entomologist's pin and a length of wire, simulated a flea bite. He discovered that the dog's hind leg would instantly scratch the appropriate area, and that it did so in a regular rhythm. It will probably not surprise the reader to learn that there are different kinds of reflexes. Sherrington's experiment demonstrated the existence of what is now known as a spinal reflex, one in which the movement is sorted out between a nerve cell in the body and one in the spinal cord, without involving the brain. Sherrington saw the reflex as the basic nervous action governing all functions in the nervous system. This may be true, in the sense that programs may be built up from sets of reflexes, but probably today most

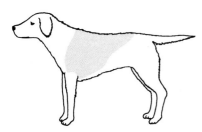

THE DISCONNECTED BRAIN
The area of skin (shown in grey) where Sherrington's dog could still scratch although its spinal cord had been cut, thus severing connection with the brain.

scientists would not agree wholeheartedly with Sherrington. Though they are all looking at the same nervous system, British neuro-scientists have tended to conceptualize, following Sherrington, in terms of reflexes, while German and American neuro-scientists have tended to conceptualize in terms of programs. Both would at least agree that reflexes are a component of movement.

One of the reasons why the reflex is an immensely useful device is because it is so fast. The knee jerk takes about a twenty-fifth of a second to operate, but a much faster one is the vestibular ocular reflex (VOR), an imposing name for the mechanism which enables us to look straight ahead even though our bodies may be moving. We all know that it is possible to fix our gaze on a point while at the same time turning our head, and so keep track of things while we ourselves are on the move. The speed of the VOR is very fast, about one one-hundredth of a second, and it needs to be, because if we had to 'think' about these reflexes they would not operate at fast enough speeds to enable us to carry out our intentions in the world. It is as if for most of our lives we are on auto-pilot; and that seems very close to the conduct of a machine.

PLANNING A MOVEMENT

It seems, then, that movements, even very precise movements, are generated unconsciously for the most part. Some rather complex movements, like walking, seem to be generated in the spinal cord; some are learned 'programs' stored in the brain; some are reflex, built into the connections of the nerve-cells. Most of our voluntary movements have all three components; but we must also be able to generate a plan for the initiation of a voluntary movement. How do we do that?

In his mapping of the various parts of the brain concerned with movement, Evarts said that the frontal areas of the brain deal with motivation and ideas of future actions. Are these taking place at a conscious level? If you are playing tennis, and your opponent sends an unexpected return, how do you form the idea of where to place your racket, and with what speed to return his shot so that he will miss it? You have to form a plan of campaign in a split second, surely too fast to be 'conscious' of the plan you are making. Of course, your next move will also include elements of reflex action, to stop you falling over for one thing, and elements of learned programs, which you have acquired from past experience or from your tennis trainer, if you are so fortunate. But, over and above all this, there is in your head some sort of map or model of the actions you are about to take. What do we know about these models of action? At the Massachusetts Institute of Technology, Emilio Bizzi, who is studying the brain's mechanism of movement, believes that a human's control of his movements comes from a system which is capable of novel and creative solutions to problems of movement,

A REFLEX PATHWAY
When a muscle is stretched by additional weight (*second picture*) a signal is sent to a motor cell in the spinal cord which contracts the muscle again (*third picture*). In reality, many more nerve fibres are involved.

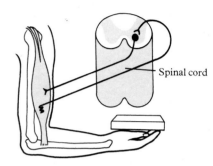

Spinal cord

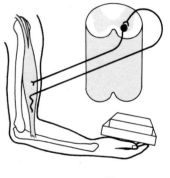

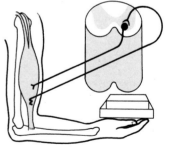

and he gives some credence to the idea that some ideal machine might be able to do it as well as we can. In his investigations into our capacity to create these models of action Bizzi finds it useful to consider the brain as if it were, in some respects at least, a computer. His explanation of the process our brain must go through in order to return the tennis ball is as follows.

> The first thing the central nervous system must compute is a representation of the external world. This is done, of course, by processing nerve signals in various visual areas in the cortex and elsewhere where a representation of the environment is created. Now from that model of the world around us, we can then compute a representation of the action; in our case, a path for the hand to take the racket to the tennis ball. Then this representation of the path of our hand has to be translated into a pattern of muscle forces, and those will actually carry the hand from its initial position to its target position.

Bizzi calls this a motor program, and all such definitions have one common theme: the notion that a program is outside the consciousness. It is mechanical, or automatic, and may be wired into the nervous system or computed or learned. But it is not a process of what we would normally describe as 'thought'.

THE INTERNAL MODEL

What is this internal representation or model of the external world, or of our movement in it, that Emilio Bizzi has described? Our internal model of *the world*, to which we relate our movements, is gained from our perception of it through our senses. Our internal model of *movement* may be a little more difficult to understand, but we all have an example literally at our fingertips. It is our signature. We all know that we will write approximately the same signature whether we do it with a pen on paper, chalk on a blackboard, or a stick in sand on the beach. Yet for each of these we use a different set of muscles. Different instructions to the muscles must come from the nervous system, but since the different combinations of different muscles result in the same signature, the internal model is not simply instructions to specific sets of muscles. Somewhere in the nervous system we formulate a model of movement which is not related to its muscular means of achievement. This is Bizzi's internal model.

A MODEL OF THE CEREBELLUM

Rodolfo Llinas of New York University has developed a theory of movement control by the brain which goes beyond theories supported by most other scientists. It is controversial, and provokes extreme reactions from its opponents. But it is a fascinating example of a concept of the brain which probably takes it as far as it is possible to go towards the machine theory.

The part of the brain which Llinas has studied most closely is the cerebellum. This is the small folded projection at the back of the brain, which plays a part in organizing and controlling movement: the output of the cerebellum appears to be almost entirely inhibitory, that is to say it prevents things rather than setting them into motion, acts as a brake rather than a motor. Thus a patient with a defect in the cerebellum finds difficulty in making smooth, co-ordinated movements. The typical neurological test is to ask the patient to place his finger on his nose, and what follows is usually a wayward deviating path for the finger through the air before it finally arrives, with a great deal of difficulty, at the nose. It seems that the cerebellum makes sure that skilled movements do not over-run; that it, as it were, sets margins beyond which movements are not allowed to go. The cerebellum, perhaps of all parts of the brain, seems to have the most characteristics which are associated with the workings of a computer.

Because of the devoted work of many scientists the structure of the cerebellum is rather well understood – better, perhaps, than any other part of the brain. Its fundamental anatomy was set out as early as 1888 by the Spanish neuroanatomist Santiago Ramon y Cajal. Since then the function of the various cells and cell types in the cerebellum, and their interconnections, has been worked out in detail. The cortex of the cerebellum is folded and convoluted like the cerebral cortex, but its structure is so regular as to be almost stereotyped. It is as if it is built of a regular succession of micro-circuits, each containing half a dozen different kinds of cells, arranged and connected in the same way from section to section. Because the structure is so regular and so well known, one slice of

A PURKINJE CELL
Diagram of an output nerve cell of the cerebellum, named after a Czech neuroanatomist of the 19th century. (*Left*) a simplified form of the cell produced by a computer after careful measurement of many real cells.

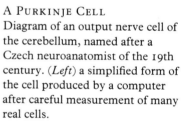

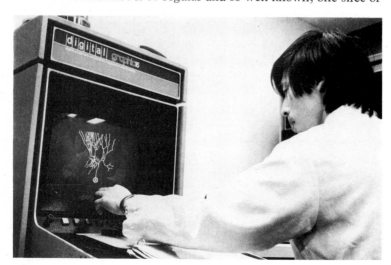

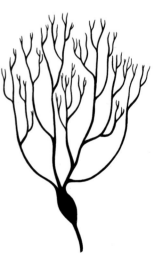

the cerebellum is much like another; it has been helpful to experimentalists who employ techniques like brain-slice physiology. In this technique the slice of brain is kept alive for many hours in a fluid and can be stimulated with micro-electrodes to produce nerve signals, thus enabling physiologists to study the processes going on inside.

Llinas has been in the forefront of such physiological research. But he no longer feels that it is an adequate way to look at cerebellar function.

> Having understood the anatomy and the electro-physiology and the circuits and the evolution and the development, we are now at a rather interesting crossroads. We must understand what the cerebellum does as a whole. Now, we're not going to understand that simply by looking at micro-electrode tracings. It doesn't exist at the tip of an electrode. So we must, by necessity, be forced to think in general terms about what the cerebellum does and how the type of experiment that we perform relates to what it actually does.

Llinas was impatient to move from collecting information to putting it together in a grand plan of brain function. He and his colleagues have done so in the most direct way, by building an artificial cerebellum. It is a working mathematical model in a computer. All available data about the function of nerve cells and nerve fibres in the cerebellum, and about the organization and function of these cells has been fed into the computer, and then mathematically combined with a theory, the tensor network theory. Llinas puts it in simpler terms:

> We have to say that the basic function of the brain relates to making an internal image of reality, and moving on the basis of that particular image. So when one considers that moving requires changing the angles of joints, you know that it must of necessity be a geometric property. There is no escaping the fact that when one wants to reach for a glass of water, one basically changes the angles of one's joints by using muscles. The other variable that is very important is time. So we combine geometry and time. Then we have a large society of nerve cells operating in unison, trying to reconstruct reality using geometry and time, and this forces us to conclude that what is happening is a geometric transformation.

By combining the physical properties, so far as they are known, of the cerebellum with this mathematical process in a computer,

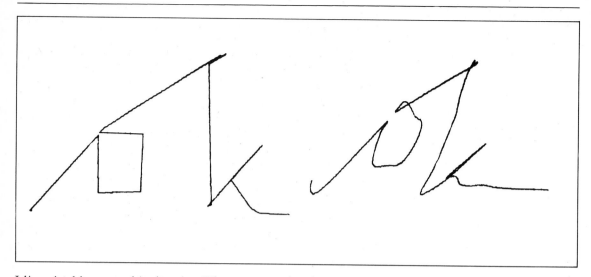

Llinas is able to test his theories. The computer has been used to produce short animated films, which show the properties of the computer's cerebellum, and the result certainly appears to be that the computer's cerebellum behaves in much the same way as a real cerebellum, albeit more crudely. Llinas is encouraged by this evidence. He also believes that it may eventually turn out that other brain structures behave in a generally similar way, though since they are less regular in form there may be many differences to be taken into account. But if just one section of the brain can be modelled in a computer in such a way that its behaviour is essentially like that of a real brain, what about the brain itself? Can it be considered a super-subtle machine? Rodolfo Llinas is not in much doubt about that.

A COMPUTER'S 'HANDWRITING'
The first picture is the geometric information given to the 'computer cerebellum'. The second is drawn by the computer using a three-jointed 'arm'. Note the apparent similarity to 'handwriting' in the second picture.

> I think when people think of machines, they think of man-made machines. A machine basically means to me any device capable of complex behaviour, and I would have no problem considering an insect, or even a lower vertebrate, a machine. As far as I'm concerned, I would consider myself a very complicated device, a very complicated machine if you like, but not very much more than that. I suppose it is a question of personal choice, and I have no quarrel with being a machine. What that says is that we may have a lot to learn about machines, that machines in principle are not silly, or incapable of the sort of things that human beings can do, loving and remembering and so forth. I know I'm an invention of my brain, I am one of the possible functional states of my brain. I seem to exist during the day, but at night, when I fall asleep 'I' disappear and yet my brain goes on in another fashion, another functional state. So I am, therefore, a functional state of my brain.

When the Plan Goes Wrong

Evidently even the consideration of movement is leading us into deep philosophical waters, which are plumbed to greater depths in the chapter on the self. At the present level, however, let us consider the riddle posed by disorders of movement, some of the states in which, Dr Llinas would no doubt say, the machinery goes wrong. Parkinson's Disease provides some awkward questions, but it may also help us find some answers.

Many of us will unfortunately suffer from Parkinson's Disease as we grow older, for it is widespread. It has several symptoms, the one with which we are most familiar being the characteristic tremor. (It was once known as the shaking palsy.) Only about seventy per cent of sufferers from Parkinson's Disease have tremor, but most of them have pronounced stiffness of the limbs, even when the muscles are at rest. Patients also have difficulty with their posture, and have a tendency to stumble or fall; but the most revealing of the symptoms is akinesia, which basically means that the patient has difficulty in initiating a movement, which also tends to take him longer to carry out than normal.

One of the most celebrated experts on Parkinson's Disease is Professor David Marsden of the Institute of Psychiatry in London. One of the reasons why Parkinson's Disease is so interesting to us is that it is a disease of the brain, but it shows itself in problems of movement. Professor Marsden described the disease to us:

> The muscles themselves are normal, the nerves supplying the muscles are normal, the spinal cord and local mechanisms for controlling muscles are entirely normal, and even the more sophisticated motor mechanisms coming from the brain itself are capable of functioning normally. Somebody with Parkinson's Disease, given a big enough stimulus, can leap into action in an amazing way. The classical example is the patient who finds difficulty crossing the road, who may be very slowly cruising across when suddenly a car horn goes, and he races to the opposite side. But when he hits the pavement he can't walk again. So the basic mechanism is there, it's the starter motor that won't work.

We have seen earlier that walking is a largely automatic process, run by a program or by pattern generators. Does David Marsden think that the program has been in some way damaged?

> The patient with Parkinson's Disease has great difficulty in starting to walk, and you could say that this is simply a question of not being able to engage the program for

walking. But unfortunately even when he tries to walk the program doesn't seem to be working that well either. So I don't think it's just simply a defect in being able to pull out the program. I think the programs, too, become blurred by the illness.

Marsden also believes that there is some obstacle between the patient's intention to move and his ability, somewhere in that rather grey area of will and desire. 'Patients will typically say that they know exactly what they want to do, and they're keen to do it, but they just can't get their muscles to obey the dictates of their will. It's as though there is some block between their conscious desire and their motor apparatus.'

COPING WITH PARKINSON'S DISEASE

A few years ago, the actor Terry Thomas developed Parkinson's Disease, and in his mews house in London he described to us what the symptoms were like, and how it affected him.

I didn't know anything about Parkinson's, like most people, so I didn't know what I was going to get. I knew there was something wrong with me when I found I couldn't jump as high as I usually could, and I lost my joie de vivre, which is an English word meaning gusto. My left hand started bouncing about all over the place, and also I felt very depressed. If you've got a wonky hand and you're depressed, you've got a wonky hand and you're depressed: but if somebody tells you that you've got Parkinson's Disease it starts a new thing altogether. . . .

Sometimes it's almost impossible to walk, and other times I can walk very well. A few months ago, I suddenly felt like dancing. It's a very weird thing. Sometimes I don't sleep very well, and when I wake up I get a piece of chocolate, and I have to go through a door from my bedroom into the kitchen where the chocolate is. One night, coming to the door, I couldn't get through it and I had to force my way through it. It was as if one's feet were glued to the ground. I've tried tricks like dancing through, and sometimes it's worked. And then one says that that's settled, and the next day you try to do it and you're falling about. I feel that I'm something like a giraffe with a couple of vertebrae that have been kicked in or something.

Obviously, Terry Thomas has kept more than a spark of his sense of humour. His courage in the face of the crippling effects of

Parkinson's Disease was evident, and he was very concerned that the world should understand the problems patients have, and not avoid them. Understanding, in the widest sense, can help to alleviate, and may lead to a cure.

MESSAGES THAT PASS THE GAP

Nerve cells do not form a continuous network. As microscopes improved during the nineteenth century and staining procedures also improved, it became possible to see the points at which one nerve fibre connected with another. There are many many such junctions. It looked, even through the microscopes of the 1890s, as if there might be some form of gap between the cells. It was Sherrington who christened this gap 'the synapse', derived from the Greek word for a handclasp. Sherrington had deduced the existence of the synapse, partly from the evidence of microscopy, but partly because he had become convinced that different cells had different functions, and that there must therefore be some essential discontinuity between them. His deduction proved to be true, and today synapses can be seen quite clearly through the electron microscope, which was, of course, not available in Sherrington's lifetime.

Nerve impulses travel along nerve fibres as an electrical wave, but they cross the synapse by means of chemicals. One side of the synapse stores these signal-carrying chemicals in tiny bags, called vesicles. When the nerve is electrically excited, these vesicles swarm to the membrane, penetrate it, and release their contents across the synaptic gap. When the molecules of messenger chemical, or neuro-transmitter, reach the membrane of the cell with which the first cell is communicating, they cause the second cell in turn to become electrically excited and the nerve signal is passed through the second cell and its fibres once again in an electrical fashion. If there is an insufficient quantity of the messenger chemical, or neuro-transmitter, the second cell will not fire. This appears to be the cause of Parkinson's Disease. By examining the brains of patients with Parkinson's Disease who have died, it was discovered that part of the basal ganglia, one of the regions concerned with movement, was deficient in the compound known as dopamine, a neuro-transmitter somewhat akin to adrenalin. The dopamine appeared to be absent from a part of the basal ganglia which is normally rich in the chemical, the region called the *substantia nigra* (black substance). The obvious remedy of supplying more dopamine was not practicable, because dopamine cannot be fed to the patient and arrive in the brain. But a substance was available – having been isolated years before – which the patient could take orally, and which would be converted in his brain to dopamine. This was L-DOPA. Sure enough, when patients were given L-DOPA, their symptoms were dramatically relieved. As doctors have become more familiar with this drug, they have discovered that it has a number of undesirable side-effects and that other drugs may need to be taken to counter them. The exact dosage of L-DOPA given to the patient is also important: one patient may need more than another, and a patient may need more as his disease progresses. L-DOPA, it should be remembered, is not a cure for Parkinson's Disease but a chemical which will relieve its symptoms. Its undesirable effects arise because dopamine is lacking, as far as we know, only in the area of the substantia nigra; but the drug L-DOPA, of course, sends dopamine all over the brain and not just to the target area. As yet, it is impossible to administer the drug in such a way that it only goes to the substantia nigra, but the relief of symptoms is so marked that most patients are willing to put up with the side-effects.

A DEFECT OF WILL?

The Parkinson's patient, then, has this strange inability to translate his intention into movement. And we can point to the substantia nigra, in the basal ganglia, as the site of the obstacle. Is the substantia nigra, therefore, the place in the brain where we convert intention into movement? Is it a particular gateway in the brain's computer mechanism? The pathway, perhaps, between an internal model and its execution? Even the route that free-will takes?

Unfortunately, like most brain structures, the basal ganglia seem to have a number of functions. They are connected, for example, with emotional disturbances in some diseases. Although we can infer some of their functions by studying nerve pathways leading into and out of them, we cannot yet be very specific about their exact role in the great drama of the brain. When we do, we shall no doubt discover that they are concerned with many more aspects of brain activity than those which are at present detectable.

It is fascinating that a Parkinson's patient can galvanize himself into movement, or be galvanized into movement, by psychological means. Terry Thomas mentioned that he could dance through a door but he couldn't walk through, and Professor Marsden mentioned that a Parkinson's patient can run across the road if he feels danger threatening. In the same way, patients who have difficulty in taking a first step sometimes find that they can do so if they say to themselves not 'I will take a step' but 'I will reach that piece of furniture'. This may, perhaps, utilize some other brain mechanism than the one normally used for the transition from intention to action. Emotional arousal, perhaps, enables the movement to be made. There seems to be a connection between psychology and movement which might not have been expected. If the action of the drug L-DOPA is only to mend a missing connection, as it were, but the disease still has these curious implications perhaps linked with will and emotion, the hypothesis

L-DOPA BECOMES DOPAMINE
The molecule of the inert L-DOPA is shorn of a few carbon, oxygen and hydrogen atoms by an enzyme to become the neurotransmitter, dopamine.

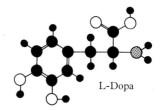

L-Dopa

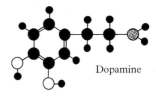

Dopamine

that the brain is essentially an incredibly complex machine, but still a machine, seems to be further reinforced. How can breaking a connection interfere with such a human attribute as 'will'? And is there any other way of re-making the connection?

BRAIN TRANSPLANTS IN PROSPECT

Anders Bjorklund, whose laboratory is in the University of Lund, in Sweden, has been active in brain science for many years and has been associated with a number of developments, especially in the field of neuro-chemistry, and particularly with dopamine. He has produced what he believes to be a model form of Parkinson's Disease in rats by destroying the dopamine cells in their brains. A rat with large-scale dopamine cell loss does show a condition not unlike that of a patient with advanced Parkinson's Disease. It is quite unresponsive and unable to initiate movement, and certainly looks very sick. But if the rat is given L-DOPA, it will regain most of its previous function. Partly on the basis of such experiments, Bjorklund believes that dopamine, though it no doubt acts as a normal neuro-transmitter, also sets some kind of threshold in the brain. Without dopamine, he suggests, systems function very inadequately, and in such instances the stimulus needed for reactivating the system, therefore, must be a very profound one. (This chimes with the phenomenon previously mentioned by David Marsden: a threat of danger such as an approaching car enables the patient to move with unaccustomed speed.)

Not all Bjorklund's rats are totally inactivated. Some are damaged only on one side, and they have a characteristic movement biased towards the side on which the dopamine cells have been destroyed. This gives him a convenient method of assessing the spectacular treatment he gives them.

With the assistance of his colleagues, Bjorklund takes cells from the brain of an embryo rat and transplants them to the brain of the 'Parkinsonian' rat. It turns out that the brain is a favourable site for this kind of transplant – it does not have so severe a 'rejection' response as other organs of the body – and growth of the embryo nerve cells seems to take place without great difficulty. Originally the transplant was in the form of a tiny plug of brain tissue, but now the cells are injected into the brain as a suspension. In both methods, not only do the cells remain alive and develop, but they send fibres to targets which normal dopamine cells would seek out, despite the fact that the transplant is made in a region some distance from the damaged dopamine cells. This action of the implanted cells would be only an interesting phenomenon if it were not that they restore movement to the Parkinsonian rat! The one-sided rat begins to move quite normally again. Because movement is restored, although the transplant cells are placed in the wrong position, these experiments support Bjorklund's theory that the dopamine system sets thresholds rather than simply transmitting information; the latter would seem to require more precise implantation. The dopamine cells may activate other systems of the brain rather than relaying messages from one part of the brain to another.

It may come as a surprise to find that brain cells can regenerate. It is indeed true that, once cells have been destroyed, connections are not again made, but it is thought that it may be scar tissue that prevents the re-establishment of connections, rather than the total inability of the cell to produce new fibres. New fibres may grow, but cannot cross the scar tissue. The fibres from the transplant cells are able to find their way to the target cells, it is thought, by means of a chemical signal. The process is perhaps rather analogous to that by which a male moth finds his way to a female moth across long distances by homing in on the sex-attractant scent which the female uses. It is believed that fibres from nerve cells in the developing brain of a foetus find their route and destination by means of such chemical signals.

The temptation, then, is to anticipate an application of Bjorklund's technique and ask if it is likely that patients with Parkinson's Disease will ever be cured by means of such brain transplants. Dr Bjorklund is reluctant to make such guesses.

> It's dangerous to guess. It's to some degree science fiction because one has to remember that these experiments are much easier with rats. But it would be impossible even to imagine using human foetuses for the same purposes, even if we were sure that it would work. Going ahead too quickly may very well set back the development of the technique. This has been seen, I think, in other transplantation techniques.

Bjorklund believes that the technical problems may, in time, be overcome, but that the ethical problems are far more intractable. However, American scientists have recently announced that dopamine-containing cells from the adrenal gland have been used in similar transplantation techniques. It may be, then, that adrenal cells from the patient himself could be used to correct his symptoms of Parkinsonism. But any such technique is likely to be for the very distant future.

THE HUMAN MACHINE

We know a great many facts about how the brain enables us to move. And for the most part they do seem to suggest that this function of the brain, at least, operates like a machine, albeit a machine of such complexity and beauty that it could not be built by man in anything like the present state of his knowledge. But the systems of the brain that are responsible for our movements are also connected with many other systems responsible for other faculties of humankind. Since we need to move to attain any of our ends or desires, movement may be regarded as being the servant of some higher function, of thought, or philosophy, intellectual activity of a noble kind. Conversely, it may be that what we think of as the higher functions serve instead to refine the many movements through which we attain our goals. Our undoubted increase in intellectual capacity through evolution may have been intended to enable us to behave, that is to move and to act, more efficiently. Perhaps those 'higher' intellectual processes may also be the work of a superb machine; if so, if the human might be thought of as a wonderfully complex machine, could one have free-will? The question was put to David Marsden:

> Certainly I believe one has free-will because one can make conscious decisions. But you're really asking about the brain mechanism for making conscious decisions. The first mechanism must be the capacity to introspect one's own conscious experience and thought process, and the capacity to introspect, I believe, must have some physiological basis which will sooner or later be established. And the moment one has the ability for a machine to introspect its own workings, then it can start to sift its own stores of memories or circumstance, its own feelings, and come to conclusions as to what it would like to do at a particular instant. I don't see why a machine should not be able to do that. I don't see how — but I don't see why not.

That statement bears comparison with a view expressed over 300 years ago by René Descartes, pioneer of modern philosophy:

> To those who know how many different automata or moving machines can be made by man's industry, with the use of very few pieces, compared to the great multitude of bones, muscles, nerves, arteries, veins and other parts of an animal body, it will not seem strange to consider this body as a machine, which being made by the hands of God is incomparably better ordered, and has more admirable motions than anything which can be invented by man.

Some scientists, then, are not averse, at least in principle, to believing themselves machines. Other scientists vehemently disagree, and for most of us the question must remain open. But living machines may be different even from machines like computers; and the next chapter adds a further layer of complexity which, curiously enough, begins further back in evolution.

CHAPTER 5

FEAR

Before nervous systems had evolved, cells could communicate by chemical messages. The chemicals in our nervous system today are present in very primitive creatures, and parsimonious Nature has continued to use them for new purposes in our brains. This ancient system links our brains to our bodies, and shows that they cannot be thought of in separation. We call this linkage emotion; and of all the emotions the one we examine in this chapter is probably the most primitive: fear. But, as we shall see, fear can also help the rational brain with which we are becoming familiar.

A VERY RATIONAL FEAR

Tony Boucher stepped out – into 2500 feet of thin air. It was his first parachute jump, and in addition to a couple of parachutes he also had strapped to him a tape recorder and a heart-beat monitor. He was a guinea-pig in a simple experiment aimed at investigating the body's reaction to – and perfectly rational fear of – the prospect of falling from a very great height.

His heart-beat had been measured continuously during the period of pre-drop training – a total of thirty-six hours – and at the tense time immediately prior to the aircraft's take-off it was registering 130 beats per minute. At the instant of jumping his heart rate rose to its highest, 170 beats per minute. It began to slow as soon as his parachute opened, and did not reach 170 again even in the course of an unexpectedly hazardous landing.

A change in wind blew him towards some of the airfield buildings, a dangerous feature which had been particularly discussed in training. Instead of adopting the approved technique of manipulating the harness toggles of the parachute to change direction, Tony made a mistake and pulled the ripcord of his reserve parachute. The result was that he was blown faster in the direction of the wind, and he was fortunate to escape almost unscathed from a very close encounter with the buildings.

Ten minutes after landing, as he was describing his experience, his heart was beating almost as fast again – so that his

THE DRUG TRAIL OF THE BRAIN
These four pictures show increasing magnifications of a section of monkey's brain. It has been treated to pick out high concentrations of receptors of substances in the brain which are mimicked by drugs like opium and morphine (*see page 142*). The original microscope pictures have been processed by computer to sharpen contrast between the concentrations of receptors. Purple is low density and progressive increases are shown by blue, green, yellow, red and white respectively.
1. The whole brain
2. (*Above*) the hypothalamus (*Below*) the amygdala.
3. The base of the hypothalamus which controls output of hormones by the pituitary gland.
4. The median eminence of the hypothalamus. Note the high concentration of receptors in the red area.

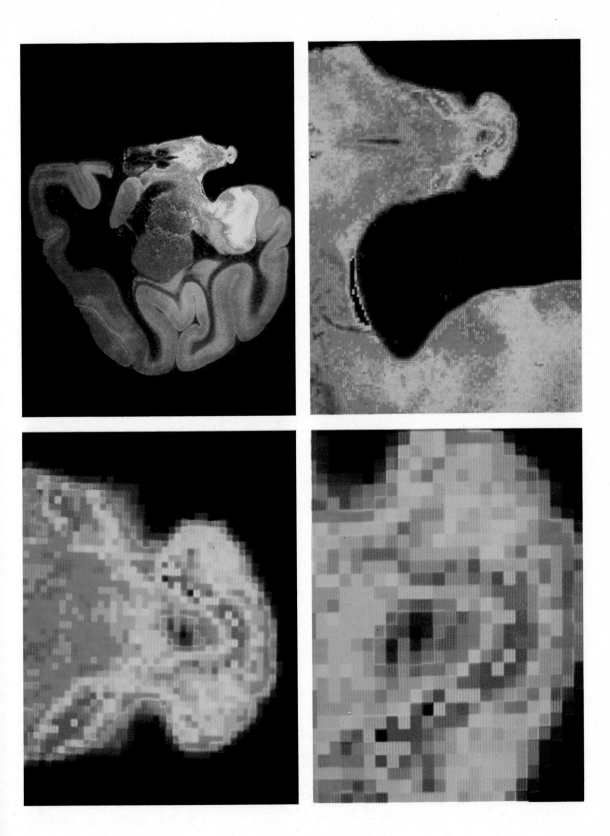

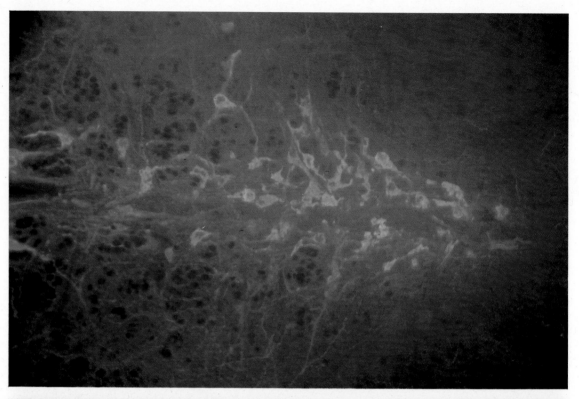

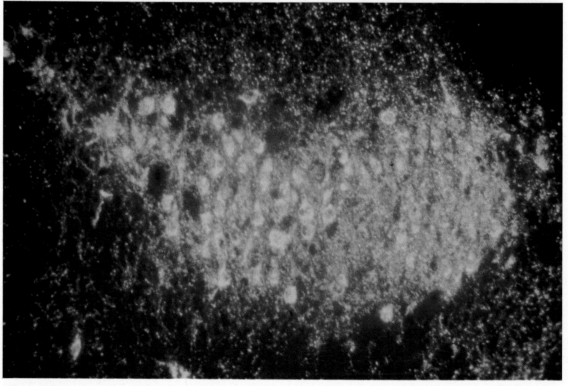

FROZEN WITH TERROR

The natural brain chemical serotonin may be responsible for the 'freezing with terror' response of someone exposed to extreme danger. (*Above*) the serotonin in these cells in the brain stem has been stained to fluoresce red under ultra-violet light.

FIGHT OR RUN

(*Below*) these cells in the brainstem contain noradrenalin which has been treated to glow green. Noradrenalin is thought to mediate the 'fight or flight' response.

FEAR OF FLYING

The record of Tony's heart-rate made by his tape-recorder. Note the highest peaks are as he leaves the plane and about ten minutes later.

re-living the experience was almost as exciting as actually having it in the first place. And the experiment provided a good example of induced fear of the most basic kind, fear for survival, fear of death.

A SPECTRUM OF FEAR

There is a spectrum of fear, ranging from mild disquiet to raging terror, and in psychological terms it is an emotion that is distinguished from anxiety, and from stress. In what follows, in an essentially biological approach, the terms fear, stress and anxiety are considered to be emotions with approximately the same physical effects, although academic scientists might not care for that simplification. (Depression, on the other hand, has different effects on the body and the brain, and does not form part of the discussion.) We all know that we would *feel* different when faced by a man with a gun, or an income-tax inspector with a final demand, but our bodies would be reacting in much the same way, and brains are only parts of the body.

The response we all have when faced with a terrifying object is what is called the 'fight or flight' response. This is just what it seems to be: if we are faced with a dangerous situation we can either fight or run away. In either case we will need more energy, and that we obtain from sugar in the blood, so our hearts beat faster to get more fresh blood to the muscles.

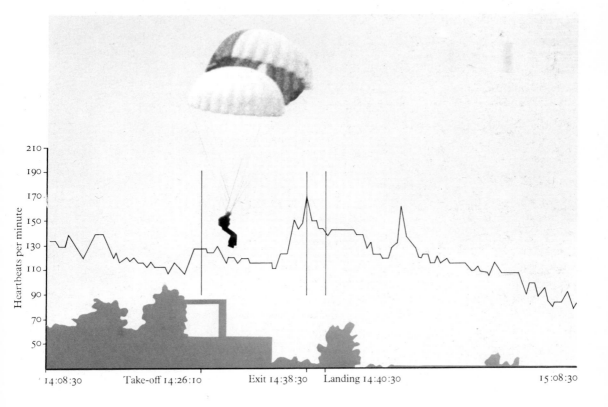

14:08:30   Take-off 14:26:10   Exit 14:38:30   Landing 14:40:30   15:08:30

The response has an obvious evolutionary value. When a gazelle sees a lion approaching, he will be prudent to run away. If it were not so, there would be fewer gazelles today. The response helps the species to survive. And the physiological response in the body of the gazelle is the same as the physiological response in the body of Tony Boucher and not very different from what is going on in the pursuing lion. Professor of Psychiatry, Isaac Marks:

> It's not clear whether what happens during intense fear is any different from what happens during intense rage . . . our hearts start beating faster, we become aware of the heart-beat, we start sweating, and our hair starts standing on end; and if it's extreme terror we might want to pass water. These are the main sensations. Then there is a whole variety of biochemical changes as well . . . these also tend to occur during rage and they might even occur during intense sexual excitement. The differences between the physiological patterns of the different emotions are less important than the similarities.

Rage, fear and sexual excitement are sometimes grouped together as 'arousal', because of their similar body reactions. The mental causes may be very different, and of course we are all perfectly aware that we *feel* different when we are enraged or sexually excited. But the underlying bodily events may be very similar. As for the brain, it is likely that, here too, the patterns are not so very different from each other. All our emotions are rooted in joint activity of body and brain, and all of them involve changes in our chemistry. In investigating such activities and changes we shall consider fear to be a model emotion.

THE CHEMISTRY OF FEAR

Otto Loewi, an Austrian scientist, won the Nobel Prize for Physiology in 1936. In 1921 he carried out the experiment for which he is famous, a demonstration which disproved the then conventional wisdom that all messages pass between nerve cells by means of electricity. Loewi was convinced that it was a chemical which stimulated the heart to change its rate of beating. Two nerves run to the heart from the brain, one of which, the vagus nerve, is responsible for slowing the heart rate, and Loewi was certain that there was a chemical component in this action.

Loewi took two frogs' hearts, kept them alive by bathing them in fluid, and stimulated the vagus nerve of the first with an electric shock. The heart, as expected, slowed. Then he took some of the fluid which had bathed the heart and added it to fluid flowing through the second heart. The second heart also slowed down. The first heart's nerve cells must have released something, a chemical, into the fluid which affected the second heart. Clearly the nerves were not acting directly, but through a 'slow-down' chemical substance, later identified as acetylcholine. The heart's 'speed-up' nerve, the accelerans, used adrenalin to achieve its effect in the frog. (It was later discovered that in most other animals the 'accelerator' chemical is noradrenalin, a close relative of adrenalin.)

The result of Loewi's experiment provides us with the first chemical connection between the fear response and the nervous system. The complete picture is more complex, however, and involves the concept of the autonomic nervous system. Earlier in the book we provided descriptions of the central nervous system and the peripheral nervous system. They are essentially definitions related to location. The autonomic nervous system, a classification by function, comprises those parts of the other two systems which have connections with the heart and many of the other internal organs. It uses acetylcholine and noradrenalin as its transmitters.

THE AUTONOMIC NERVOUS SYSTEM

The sympathetic system is mostly arousing, and the parasympathetic system is calming: sympathetic nerves accelerate the heart and parasympathetic nerves slow it. There are exceptions, however, and in extreme fear, for example, parasympathetic nerves cause the bladder and bowels to discharge.

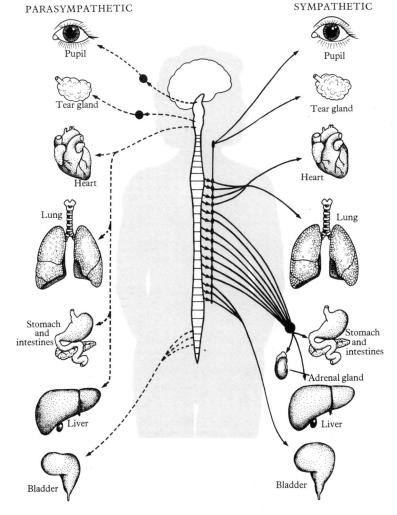

PARASYMPATHETIC · SYMPATHETIC

Pupil · Pupil
Tear gland · Tear gland
Heart · Heart
Lung · Lung
Stomach and intestines · Stomach and intestines
Adrenal gland
Liver · Liver
Bladder · Bladder

These are the substances that cross the synapse, or gap, at the connections between one nerve cell and another and so carry the signal along a nerve from, say, the brain to the heart. But adrenalin and noradrenalin are hormones, released by the adrenal gland. The role of such hormones in the bloodstream is more general than the specific nerve-transmission effects of themselves and of chemicals like acetylcholine. But it is still directed towards the same end, and maintains a state of physical arousal that follows the first nerve signals that speed up the heart. (That the body and the brain can use one chemical for a number of different purposes is a parsimony which has sometimes confused experimenters, and still does.)

STRESS AND THE FEAR REACTION

Near the beginning of this chapter we mentioned that stress, an emotional state, could produce the same physical reaction as fear. Let us look at one or two instances of physical arousal generated by mental stress.

Most of us may find mental arithmetic boring, though few of us would perceive it objectively as threatening. But Dr Fred Imms at RAF Chessington can demonstrate that mental stress of this kind is as threatening, to judge from physical effects, as the real danger of a lion or a parachute jump. Dr Imms carried out a controlled test in which his subject, who was lying down in physically non-stressful circumstances, was asked to subtract seven from nine hundred and ninety nine successively and continuously. The subject's heart-rate was monitored, and rose from 75 at the beginning of the session to 114 at the end. The state of a body's preparedness for fight or flight can be displayed on a device called a plethysmograph, which is attached to a subject's leg, and measures its volume of blood. During the mental arithmetic the blood volume of the monitored subject rose markedly, showing that, although he was lying down, his body was preparing for instant flight – just like the gazelle pursued by the lion. So pure mental stress can induce the physical characteristics of real danger, and these may be quite undesirable, particularly if the physical reactions interfere with a skilled performance.

Our second experiment in the physical effects of stress was slightly more involved, and was based on the effect of stage-fright in musicians. The experiment was devised by Dr Ian James of the Royal Free Hospital, London.

We found six young violinists and took them to a London concert hall, where we filmed them in rather stressful conditions. The film crew was primed to be as unlike its normal self as possible: cold, dictatorial and unhelpful. In addition, Ian James arranged for a music assessor to be present to comment on the performance of the six violinists. There were two sessions. In the morning, each violinist played a Bach piece, specially selected because it begins

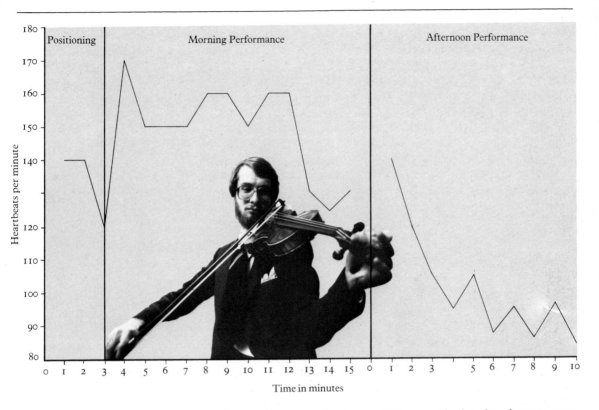

PETER'S HEART RATE
The morning performance shows a violinist's heart beating at a peak of 170, and remaining at 150 or so most of the time. In the afternoon after taking beta-blockers, his heart rate settles at about 90.

with a very long sustained note. This was calculated to show up any tremor, or any lack of skill due to sweaty hands, both bodily responses to stress or to fear. Then some of the violinists were given a drug, while the others were given an inert placebo. It was quite evident in the second session that the performance of those subjects who had played badly in the morning was materially improved by the drug. And, in addition, they felt less anxious.

The drug, a 'beta-blocker', is normally used to treat some heart conditions. It was invented as a result of research that followed from Loewi's discovery of the chemical control of the heart-rate. The effect of the beta-blocker drug taken by the violinists was to stop the action of adrenalin. Adrenalin has its effect on nerve cells because its molecules fit into other molecules called receptors on the cell membrane (in our example, on cells in the violinist's heart). These receptors may be thought of as a keyhole and the adrenalin molecule as a key. For adrenalin there are two types of receptor keyholes, the alpha and the beta, and when the adrenalin key fits in the beta receptor keyhole it accelerates the heart. It also dilates blood vessels in muscle and skin, and relaxes the muscles of the bladder and intestine. Many of our responses to danger or stress are switched on through such receptors.

The beta-blocker, as its name implies, blocks the beta receptor and when it is stuck fast will prevent adrenalin having its usual effect. Thus it helped to block the physical effects on the violinists which interfered with their performances. Curiously, it also reduced the *feeling* of anxiety. The violinists noticed this. Said one, 'The second time I was less nervous both physically as well as mentally. My bowing was a lot better and that was completely under control the second time and I felt much happier generally.' Another said, 'Certainly the beta-blockers made you relax more mentally and physically.' Another of the violinists made the point, though, that it was not only the pills which made a difference between the first and second time. 'The second time I didn't feel so nervous of the start. I started more cleanly, which may have been to do with the pills, or it may have been also to do with the fact that I was more at home in the surroundings and more used to the acoustics. But I think a combination of the two, really.' The demonstration of the effects of beta-blockers was certainly convincing, but a warning is necessary. Since the drug is a powerful one, it should never be taken without a doctor's advice.

Even if we did not know it was a hormone, most of us have heard of adrenalin as a substance found in greater quantities in the bloodstream at times of physical arousal. We've all heard someone say, 'That gets the adrenalin flowing.' In recent experiments, adrenalin turns out to have an effect on what we think of as a mental function, memory. It may even explain, as we shall see, why our novice parachutist, Tony Boucher, made his mistake.

Dr James McCaugh, at the University of California at Irvine, has shown that when rats are given an injection of adrenalin in the body, not the brain, after learning a simple task, their memory is affected. The time and quantity of the application is critical; very simply, just the right amount will strengthen the memory, too much will cause memory loss, or amnesia. Adrenalin given thus cannot reach the brain, so, in some way we do not yet fully understand, body hormones affect the brain, as well as vice versa. In Tony's case, it may have been that, because he was very physically aroused, too much adrenalin (or some related hormone) caused him to forget, and release his second parachute, with dire consequences. Properly tuned hormone release and consequent arousal, though, may well be a mechanism that helps us learn the right response to a danger.

THE PARALYSIS OF FEAR

We have seen how, in response to messages from the brain, the body's chemistry, by the means of adrenalin release, then stimulates the body into action – fight or flight – to counter a threat. That is not the only physical reaction in face of real or imagined danger, because there is quite a different response, captured in the phrase 'frozen with terror'. In the example we shall give, we look at the case of the victim of a phobia – a condition which we shall explore subsequently – but the reaction of paralysis is far from confined to irrational fears or imagined threats.

Beverley Sadler from Enfield is an arachnophobe, which means that she has a fear of spiders. But in Beverley's case 'absolute terror' might be a better description. She tells of her fear, of the classic sensations of phobia that she experiences, and how on one occasion she found a spider in her bedroom, which induced a paralysis of terror:

> I've always been frightened of them . . . I break out in a cold sweat, my legs start to shake, and I go to jelly virtually, and I've just got to get away from it. I feel as if I am going to faint and I just feel hot and cold, and I want to cry. . . . One time the spider was on a book on the bed and I couldn't go past the bed or the book or move the book to move the spider. I just stood transfixed in a corner and that's where I stayed for three hours.

This seems to be a rather extreme example of the phenomenon of being 'frozen with terror', or 'rooted to the spot'. How does it happen? The explanation may be a chemical one. Dr Gordon Gallup of the University of New York at Albany is examining a particular chemical, and a similar effect produced in animals by that chemical.

Gallup demonstrates what is popularly called 'animal hypnosis' with the help of a pet rooster called Henry. He places Henry gently on his back, holds him for a few seconds, then slowly removes his hand, and the rooster remains quite motionless, apparently hypnotized. Henry's eyes remain open, but glazed, and he languidly extends each leg. Says Gallup, 'It turns out that, in spite of the superficial similarities between animal hypnosis and human hypnosis, the evidence strongly suggests that this is not a hypnotic reaction, in fact that it's more probably a fear reaction.' Gallup has found that the same phenomenon also occurs in insects, crustacea, reptiles, and mammals, even primates. Henry is brought out of his trance by a snap of Gallup's fingers, and is apparently quite untroubled by the experience. Normally the immobility lasts for only a few minutes, but it can be extended by various means, and Gallup's laboratory record currently stands at about five hours forty-five minutes. To achieve such a long period of immobility Gallup places a stuffed hawk near Henry. Even a pair of glass eyes, on the end of two sticks, like hawks' eyes, will achieve the same result. But Gallup wanted to go further, and he proceeded, like Loewi, to test a chemical hypothesis.

Gallup suspected that the effect might be mediated by a neuro-transmitter, serotonin. This chemical, like the adrenalin which influences the heart, is one of the messenger chemicals which carry nerve signals across synapses, including those in the brain. Gallup did controlled experiments in which he injected half of his experimental chickens with the raw material from which the brain

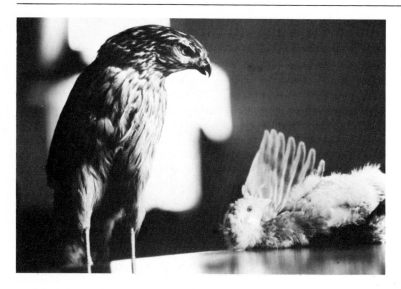

A CHICKEN PLAYS POSSUM
One reaction to fear which may be
controlled by the serotonin
pathways in the brain.

makes serotonin, tryptophan. Sure enough, the injected birds
stayed in their trance-like states for longer than the birds which had
not been given the tryptophan. Other experiments confirmed that
the response was prolonged by the treatment, and this points to the
involvement of the chemical serotonin. Not only is the body's fight
or flight response switched on by chemicals, so is the 'frozen with
terror' response; but we don't know as yet how the mechanism
works.

Gallup believes that the immobility may be part of a defence
mechanism. He cites the case of the proverbial cat and mouse
where, following initial capture, frequently the cat will back off and
wait for the mouse to move. If the mouse fails to move, the
probability of additional attack is reduced. 'Maybe not only
possums play possum.' And one of Gallup's collaborators believes
that a similar effect may occur in cases of rape, where the victim
often ceases to struggle. Certainly, it is tempting to hypothesize that
Beverley's reaction to the spider in her bedroom was controlled by
serotonin circuits in her brain. The chemicals act there as well as in
the rest of the body.

The experiment with the chickens shows also that emotions
such as fear are sometimes derived from built-in mechanisms. The
chickens, including Henry, which were the subjects of Gallup's
experiments, had never seen a hawk, much less a pair of
disembodied eyes, yet they reacted to it appropriately. The fear of
hawks or hawk-like objects had been with them since they were
eggs; it was handed down to them by their parents. Some of our
human fears may also be genetic in origin, but others are learned
during life. Both inherited and learned fear, though, have much the
same effect on the chemistry of our bodies, and of our brains. We do
not know whether phobias like Beverley's are due to inheritance, or
to a past, forgotten experience.

ASPECTS OF PHOBIA

Phobics commonly find it difficult to discuss their phobia with other people. In the first place, to talk about it brings the dreaded object to mind. In the second place, despite all assurances to the contrary, they are convinced that they are the only person in the world who has this uncontrollable terror. And they are frightened of appearing comic or ridiculous.

What about Beverley's fear of spiders? Undeniably the spider is a powerful symbol of horror. In Freudian analysis it represents some morbid sexual problem. But in most countries, and certainly in Great Britain, there is no sensible reason to be afraid of spiders. Some people, however, are literally frozen by terror in the presence of just one of the creatures, for this is a common phobia, along with morbid terror of birds, or of open spaces. It is by no means limited to those of fragile constitution or feeble mind.

Beverley's fear of spiders affects her in just the same way as the fear of battle affects soldiers, or as rational or irrational fears and anxieties affect all of us at one time or another. It is a response which involves the brain and the body, and the two responses cannot be separated. But it is not easy, or ethical, to measure the response of the human brain directly by inserting electrodes or pipettes into a patient's head; so the bodily response, which can be to a great degree equated with the brain response, is extremely valuable to the researcher, because it can be measured.

Which takes us back to our intrepid parachutist, a human being under stress who then received a severe dose of fear. Was Tony Boucher's fear the same sort of fear as Beverley Sadler's phobia? Professor Isaac Marks has made a particular study of fear:

> I suppose a normal fear like parachuting and an abnormal fear like the spider phobia are very similar. The experience is almost indistinguishable. What is different is the trigger. Nearly all of us would be terrified of parachuting, at least in the beginning, but very few of us would be absolutely paralysed with fear in the face of a spider.

TREATING A PHOBIA

Our spider phobic, Beverley, heard Professor Marks on the radio describing a treatment for phobics like herself. She rang up the radio station, and made arrangements with Marks to go to his clinic for treatment. It was a considerable ordeal for Beverley, which involved progressively more intimate exposure to the symbol of her horror, the spider. She began by looking at the picture of a spider – even that made her extremely anxious and uncomfortable – and then went on to hold the picture; then she inspected, touched and eventually picked up a dummy spider. All these stages were achieved by degrees of reluctance, but with the phobic symptoms just under control.

The next step was for her to touch a dead spider, which she eventually managed notwithstanding her clear physical discomfort. And the last act in her first therapy session, directed with sympathetic firmness by Dr Raja Ghosh, was to touch a live spider in a glass dish. That took some doing, but after a number of trial efforts she succeeded. Beverley's relief at the end of the session was obvious, but so was her pride in her achievement. She viewed her next session with great apprehension, but in the event it took only a few minutes to have a middle-sized spider running over her hand.

Professor Marks ascribes the success of this apparently simple therapy to its direct approach. The subjects are persuaded to confront their fear until the fear dies down. It owes little to the consultational-psychological approach, the search for the origins of phobias in different kinds of conflicts. Marks feels that people who in the past adopted such techniques were trying to be too clever. Marks was hopeful, though a little sceptical, about possible future drug treatment. 'It's possible that as our knowledge about the brain improves we'll be able to make the exposure treatment even more efficient than it is at the moment, or perhaps do away with it altogether. There may even be simpler ways of getting over the fear. If we knew more about the biochemistry involved we might be able to use a magic pill, though nothing like that is in sight.'

Although Professor Marks is concerned chiefly to help his patients, and no drug therapy is yet successful in curing phobias, he is well aware that biochemistry must be involved in the therapy, and that the exposure treatment is in some way altering Beverley's chemical reactions to the object of her phobia. At one level, it may be that her arousal is just enough to release the right amount of adrenalin to let her learn that spiders are harmless, even if touched or handled. But there are other chemical processes going on in her brain about which we are only beginning to learn. They concern chemical messengers, like those used in the nerves running to the heart which speed it up or slow it down.

THE PATHWAYS OF FEAR

Not all nerve cells, and not all brain cells, use the same chemical messengers, or neuro-transmitters. Certainly acetylcholine and noradrenalin are used, as is serotonin, and there are others. One chemical may be used for different purposes in different places, and chemical pathways in the brain can be traced. The pathways which seem to be associated with fear and the other emotions pass through a number of brain structures, among the most important being the hypothalamus, the thalamus, the hippocampus and the amygdala. While all these structures have a multiplicity of functions that we do not fully understand, they are each in some way connected with

BEVERLEY'S THERAPY

At stage 1, Beverley's pulse was 100. At stage 2, while holding the picture it was 110. The toy spider (3) gave a pulse of 100, as did the dead spider (4). Handling the dead spider (5) made her pulse rise to 110, and watching a live one (6) raised it to 120. When Dr Ghosh handled the live spider (7) Beverley's pulse was 100. Handling it herself (8) gave a reading of 110. After each session her pulse-rate dropped to about 75.

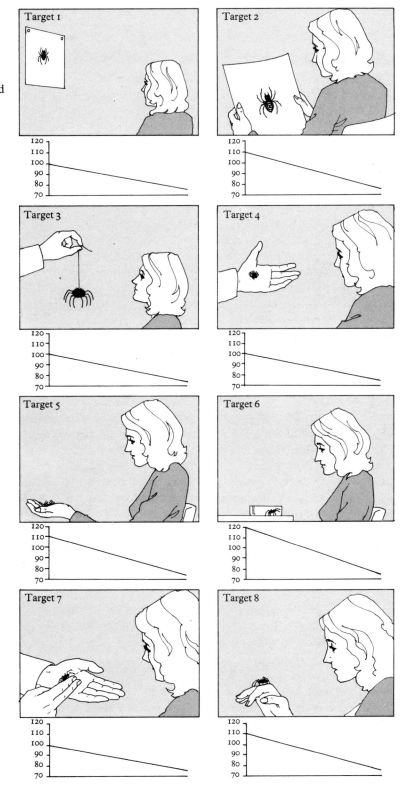

Target 1

Target 2

Target 3

Target 4

Target 5

Target 6

Target 7

Target 8

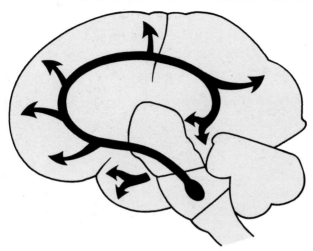

THE SEROTONIN CIRCUIT
Nerve-cells in the brain stem send
out serotonin fibres to the
emotional areas of the limbic
system as well as to other parts of
the cortex. It is associated with
temperature control and sleep.

emotion. Thus stimulation of the amygdala can cause aggressive behaviour. The hypothalamus, apart from being concerned with body temperature and appetite, regulates the pituitary gland, which in its turn governs the secretions of the important glands of the body: the ovaries and testes, the thyroid and the adrenals. The thalamus is both the junction and the integrator of circuits from many parts of the brain, including the cortex; and the hippocampus is connected with memory, so that past experience and emotion can be connected.

The chemical systems of the brain and of the nervous system in the rest of the body are closely interwoven. One of the most carefully observed has been the noradrenalin system in the brain. (Noradrenalin, remember, is the neuro-transmitter used in the 'speed-up' nerves running to the human heart.) This has for years been one of the principal preoccupations in Floyd Bloom's laboratory, in the Salk Institute in California. There is a tradition in the Salk Institute (founded by Jonas Salk, the inventor of the first vaccine for poliomyelitis) of trying to communicate scientific information to the public. Floyd Bloom embraces this tradition wholeheartedly, even though his subject of neuro-chemistry is one of the most difficult to express in layman's language. Bloom believes that it is reasonable to look for brain circuits connected with emotions, though he would not agree that the noradrenalin circuit, which he is examining, is simply an anxiety circuit. He has been studying a part of the brain stem known as the locus coeruleus, the 'blue place', where most of the brain's nerve cells using noradrenalin seem to originate. 'We can find in other parts of the brain stem the control centres of breathing, and the control of heart-rate and heart rhythm and blood pressure, and so if anxiety is on the same level as that kind of reaction then it would certainly be an appropriate area to look for a centre of brain activity to which we attribute the feeling of anxiety. But of course the activity of that centre may not be the cause, or the only cause, of our feeling anxious.'

THE NORADRENALIN CIRCUIT
This covers much the same brain
regions as the serotonin circuit (*see
diagram on page 138*). It is
concerned with arousal and with
dreaming sleep.

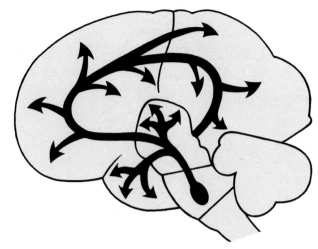

But if the locus coeruleus does affect anxiety, how does the
action of a chemical like noradrenalin make us feel anxious? Does
Bloom think it simply passes messages, or is there a particular
quality to these messages?

> At one level we can say that noradrenalin looks like an
> ordinary transmitter that makes other cells go slower,
> but when we analyse the mechanism it doesn't just make
> them go slower. It also changes the blood flow to that
> part of the brain, and changes the way oxygen moves
> from the blood to the cells that are burning carbo-
> hydrates to make energy, to make them respond to the
> signals that are coming in. It is really looking after a very
> complicated series of events. So we believe that the
> noradrenalin system is, in a California word, holistic; it
> changes several aspects of the function of the cells that
> are receiving its messages and allows them to respond
> more appropriately to what's coming into them.

Bloom has a less scientific way of giving the same message.

> One way to look at it, perhaps, is like the foot-pedals on
> the piano: you can play the same melody, but when you
> put your foot on one of the pedals, you will make your
> music sound much more beautiful or make the notes last
> much longer, and that to me is something like what the
> noradrenalin system does. It modifies how the messages
> come across.

Bloom and his colleagues are mapping the noradrenalin pathways
that extend from the locus coeruleus through the brain. The
pathways include the parts of the brain (hypothalamus, hippocampus and amygdala) that many scientists believe may be

associated with a feeling of anxiety or of fear. Eventually their map of the noradrenalin circuit will be a three-dimensional one, generated by a computer from thousands of micro-photographs.

Bloom is at pains to stress the complexity of this system and to disclaim any present giant steps in understanding. This must be built up of a multiplicity of laboriously acquired facts.

> It's very easy to make a simple hypothesis that would say noradrenalin is the transmitter of anxiety, because a drug that depletes the brain of noradrenalin changes the animal's apparent anxiety. But it's very difficult to go into the brain and say, step by step, this is how that stimulus made the animal anxious, because at step forty-seven the information got to the locus coeruleus, which then spoke to the cerebral cortex, which then spoke to the hypothalamus; and at step fifty-six the animal appears to be anxious by his behaviour and his facial gestures or whatever. There are very few things that we can come even close to understanding in the way of a real programme of events, and be able to attribute to each step of that programme the involvement of a particular neuro-transmitter chemical. It is a goal to which we all eminently aspire, but we can't do it at the moment.

Just as the noradrenalin circuit clearly has something to do with anxiety, but its role is not clear, some anxiety states can be relieved by drugs and some cannot. Phobia is not a disability which can, in the long term, be relieved by drug therapy. Professor Marks believes that other therapies will work better:

> We know that sedative drugs such as diazepam (Valium), barbiturates, and also alcohol, can give one Dutch courage for a little while as long as one has the drug or the alcohol inside one's system. One is then able to face the fear situation much better. But the problem is that as soon as the effect of the drug or the alcohol wears off, after only a few hours, then I'm afraid the Dutch courage disappears along with it.

Changing the Chemistry

The number of phobics in our society, though there are more than any of us suspect, is not very large. But there are many more people who suffer from anxiety of a more generalized kind, perhaps brought on by the ordinary stressful situations of life – work, family, money – to which a few people will always succumb. For them, relief is possible through the benzodiazepine drugs, of which the best known is perhaps Valium. The benzodiazepine drugs have

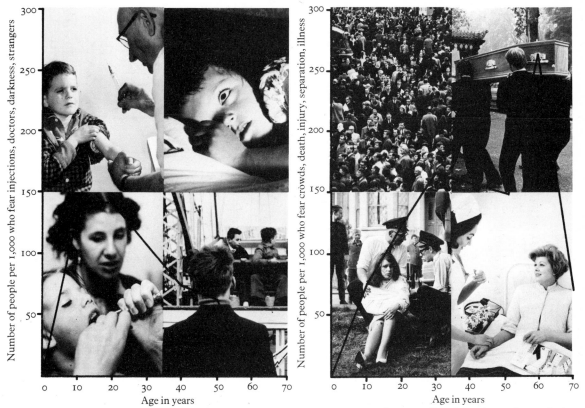

The y-axis of the left graph reads: Number of people per 1,000 who fear injections, doctors, darkness, strangers (300, 250, 200, 150, 100, 50). The x-axis reads: Age in years (0, 10, 20, 30, 40, 50, 60, 70).

The y-axis of the right graph reads: Number of people per 1,000 who fear crowds, death, injury, separation, illness (300, 250, 200, 150, 100, 50). The x-axis reads: Age in years (0, 10, 20, 30, 40, 50, 60, 70).

COMMON FEARS

Common fears associated with phobias rise to a peak at the age of 20 and then decline. Fear of doctors and darkness during childhood (*graph 1*) decline as we grow up, but fears of death and illness peak at 60 (*graph 2*).

revolutionized the treatment of generalized anxiety since their introduction in the early 1960s. In 1977 eight thousand tons were consumed in the United States. How does Valium, and the other benzodiazepine drugs, actually work on the brain? For that matter, do we know that they do have their effect on the brain? The second question is the more easily answered. A number of studies confirm that benzodiazepines are active in the brain. This can be detected in a number of regions, not just those identified earlier as being concerned with fear or anxiety symptoms. But because benzodiazepines have a number of effects besides that of relieving anxiety, including sedative, anticonvulsant, and muscle relaxant, it is to be expected that they will show activity in various parts of the brain. Their anxiety-relieving qualities, though, are those with which we are most concerned, and they are not in doubt.

As to their mode of action, the picture here is less clear. In the past, it has been established that benzodiazepines interfere with a number of the known neuro-transmitter chemicals, including serotonin and noradrenalin. At present, the neuro-transmitter which appears to be most affected by their action is GABA, gamma-amino-butyric acid. And it appears that the benzodiazepines may work through a receptor in nerve cells in the brain. That is to say, they operate as keys in a specific keyhole, much as the beta-blockers fit the beta keyhole for adrenalin.

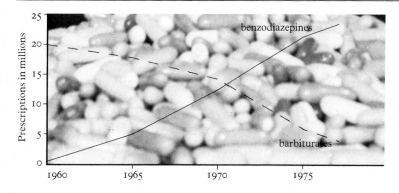

Prescriptions in millions

25
20
15
10
5
0

benzodiazepines

barbiturates

1960   1965   1970   1975

TRANQUILLIZERS
Between 1960, when
benzodiazepine drugs (which
include Librium and Valium)
became available, and 1977 they
have largely replaced barbiturates
in most countries. These figures
relate to England and Wales.

No one has yet seen a receptor, because it is simply too small to be revealed even by an electron microscope. But there has to be some molecule in the cell membrane into which active chemicals fit, the keyhole for the key. Researchers are able to establish the existence of receptors by using a suspension of brain-cell fragments, and adding to it a radio-active form of the chemical they wish to investigate – the key. After various processes, they are able to measure the radio-activity of the cell fragments and deduce the presence of receptors. It is a very time-consuming and delicate procedure, only perfected in the last few years.

The existence of the benzodiazepine receptor was established initially by two researchers in Denmark, Dr R C Squires and Dr C Braestrup. Working for a pharmaceutical company, Ferrosan, best known for its vitamin pills, Squires and Braestrup found what appears to be entirely adequate proof of the existence of the receptors.

THE FEAR SUBSTANCE

The receptor work was prompted by research done in drug addiction units in the mid-1970s which established that specific receptors exist for the opiate drugs, heroin, morphine and so forth. The next development introduced a new concept into brain chemistry. The teams who were investigating the opiates asserted that a specific receptor was not available in brain tissue to receive molecules purified from juices found only in plants, in this case the opium poppy. Their guess was that the receptors existed, but that they were already required for use by a specific substance already in the brain, for which nature had designed them. Further research did indeed find substances in the brain which have the same effect as opiates – the brain's own morphine, as it was described. Squires and Braestrup, naturally enough, hypothesized that there might also be a substance which could be the brain's own Valium.

Squires left to join another team, and Braestrup continued the research for the elusive brain chemical. The brain's own morphine had been discovered by the lengthy process of extracting chemicals from literally thousands of animals brains, an extremely expensive and time-consuming process. Braestrup, anxious to find the substance in human brains, which clearly were not available in such quantity, followed up a suggestion by Squires that it could be found in a body fluid, urine. The task of extracting chemicals from urine is hardly pleasant, and Braestrup makes it clear that he was not the most popular person in the laboratory at the time. He persuaded the staff at Ferrosan and Danish staff at the nearby hospital in Copenhagen where he also worked to collect their urine daily and pass it on to him for analysis.

> I don't know exactly how many people were involved . . . about forty at the highest. It took at least one and a half months. . . . We had to store it because we decided to wait to do the extraction until we had the whole amount. . . . When we eventually found out the way to extract it, it was awfully hard work and it was awfully smelly, but otherwise it was not all that bad. . . . It was some time until we knew we would succeed because every time we did something it was purer than it was before, but . . . the amount of material that we had was decreasing all the time. If there was too little it would be impossible to identify it.

In the earlier stages of extraction, 1800 litres of urine were reduced to a flask of a black treacly substance. At this stage it contained five thousand different chemicals. Further extraction reduced the number of chemicals to only two hundred, in a few tablespoonsful of golden liquid. At the next stage of extraction they had left perhaps one saltspoonful of clear liquid. Would this be the brain's own Valium?

It was some months before Braestrup announced the identity of the substance he had isolated. It was a betacarboline ester, a compound which is not very common in humans but, says Braestrup, quite common in some South American plants. (A tempting resemblance here to the discovery of the morphine-like chemical of a few years previously.) But did the compound have the same effects as Valium? Is it the brain's own benzodiazepine?

> That I am quite positively sure it is not. And the reason is that when we look at the way in which this compound functions in the brain we can see that while Valium is sedative in animals this compound is not sedative. It is alerting or may even induce anxiety, so we believe that this may be a compound with the opposite effect on receptors from Valium. That means that this compound may induce anxiety, or may alert people, if present in the brain.

The compound is also not quite like any substance which could be present in the brain, because the process of extraction has changed it from a natural chemical, if such there ever was. There is a great deal of controversy as to the probability of Braestrup's beta-carboline ester being a substance present in the brain at all, whether or not it has any effect on the anxiety circuits. Other researchers have produced other candidates, some of which appear equally likely. But Braestrup himself feels quite confident that, while he may not have exactly the right chemical, a closely related one will be found to be important in brain function.

But there is still the paradox that Braestrup's compound seems to have almost exactly the opposite effect to Valium. This by no means necessarily rules out its candidacy, for if there is an 'alerting compound' which the brain uses in the anxiety process, it is quite possible that Valium, occupying the same receptor, could reverse its effect. And if so, more experiments on this hypothesis could lead to a better understanding of the chemistry and to a better drug than Valium.

NEW DISCOVERIES

In the last ten years, many different chemicals have been discovered in the brain which may have many different actions. They are in different chemical groups: noradrenalin, adrenalin and dopamine, for instance are in one group; there are amino-acids, like GABA; and there are peptides, more complex structures of several amino-acids: the brain's own morphine, for example, is a peptide. We can see these chemicals glowing with their own colour signatures under ultra-violet light, forming distinct pathways in the brain tissues under inspection. But we do not yet know how they are all made, and certainly not how they act in the brain. They appear to react on one another, causing a series of events in brain cells; the chemical changes are rather like the processes in an oil refinery, where chemicals react to form new combinations; but they are certainly much more complicated than that. Very probably some of these puzzling newcomers are involved in our emotional brain circuits, and our fear reaction, but we are only just starting to understand how.

Looking at emotions, even so simple a 'gut reaction' as fear, then, gives us a window on the chemistry of the brain. At its simplest level, its chemicals function to pass messages from one cell to another. This is the business of the classical neuro-transmitter, like acetylcholine or noradrenalin. But what about the other chemicals whose actions we do not fully understand? Floyd Bloom:

> The problem that we have is that no one has yet heard directly from God what a neuro-transmitter is supposed to do. I tend to be very general about it, and I say if a

CHEMICAL KEYS
The molecules of noradrenalin and serotonin. The real properties of the molecules shown in the diagram enable them to fit receptors, or keyholes, on specific nerve cells.

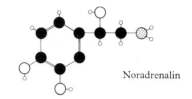

Noradrenalin

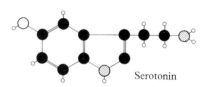

Serotonin

nerve cell has a chemical that it secretes to talk to another nerve cell, it's transmitting information. We have the two classic modes of nerve cell to nerve cell speaking: one is excitation – making it go; one is inhibition – making it stop; but then we have these nicer forms of communication which remove the sharp edges from the messages, and perhaps make them last a bit longer in memory, and perhaps do integrated things that keep the information available to be processed longer. Many people say the brain only needs an excitatory neuro-transmitter, and an inhibitory neuro-transmitter, and the rest of it is there for some inexplicable reason. For us, these inexplicable reasons are the whole basis for our research. Brain scientists are still gathering information and every time we gather a little bit of information some of the brave ones of us will try to make a theory, but they're not really fundamental theories yet. I'm hopeful that we'll be approaching that within this century. We've come an awful long way so far. We've uncovered more circuits in the last two decades than we had in all the previous history of brain research, and so we're not just understanding the continents of the brain any more, we're understanding a lot of the little villages and the byways that connect them.

Do we need drugs to abolish fear? Pain, like fear, is unpleasant, but without it we would not know when we had hurt ourselves. It is an important aid to survival. Fear and anxiety are in the same class, and a degree of anxiety is probably no bad thing, although if anxiety takes over and prevails under all conditions, then it becomes incapacitating. It then becomes necessary either that the sufferer is helped to understand his predicament or to suppress his brain's over-active propensity to anxiety. It may be that understanding and suppression are not necessarily so different. The therapy which helped Beverley Sadler cope with her fear of spiders must have operated at the level of brain chemistry. Although her treatment was behavioural and psychological, its effects must have been chemical. Her brain was adapting its own chemical circuitry. We may not yet know how, but it is an article of faith with the brain scientists that one day we shall. When we do, we shall no longer depend on the accidental discovery of useful drugs like Valium, but will be able to build precise molecules to do precise jobs for us. Or we may find ways of influencing the brain even more precisely to adjust its own chemistry, and help us to cope with our fears and anxieties.

CHAPTER 6

MADNESS

The feeling of anxiety and phobias, whether of spiders, open spaces or anything else, may severely affect one's life, possibly even dominate it, and restrict or even prevent normal work and leisure. Yet the sufferer is still fundamentally intact as an individual. The normal processes of thought and behaviour are still taking place, though perhaps with great difficulty. Anxiety is therefore what psychiatrists class as a neurosis. In the same category go other mental disorders and conditions, such as anorexia nervosa and some forms of depression.

THE INSANE ROOT

When an individual's thoughts break down so much that he or she cannot function mentally, and collapses altogether, then the psychiatrists describe the condition as a psychosis. There are varieties of psychoses, and their sub-division into those related to physical diseases (organic psychoses) and those without evident physical cause (functional psychoses) is not universally accepted, certainly not by those who believe that a disorder of the body has its reaction in the brain, and vice versa.

MENTAL DISORDERS
The brain can go wrong in as many ways as the body, so this chart only indicates the main divisions of mental disease and where schizophrenia fits in. It is the major form of insanity, and is not one but a collection of diseases.

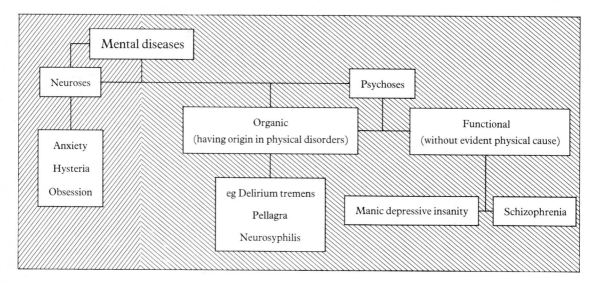

The most widespread functional psychosis is schizo-phrenia; it is the major form of madness. (The only other significant form is manic-depressive psychosis, in which it is the fierce swings of mood up or down that disrupt the sufferers' thoughts and behaviour in a dramatic way.)

Schizophrenia has been the subject of more controversy than virtually any other disease and that has often obscured the facts. Firstly, schizophrenia is madness. Secondly, one in a hundred people are affected by it; sixty thousand in Britain are in hospital because of it and a hundred thousand are in the community. Thirdly, it affects all cultures, not just those in industrialized countries. As with any disease there are individuals in whom diagnosis is difficult, some of whom are inevitably wrongly diagnosed schizophrenic, and over whom discussion and controversy understandably and rightly rage.

Indisputably schizophrenia must be the result of some change in the brain and this chapter sets the minute faults in brain chemistry that occur in the disease against the sadness and debility caused by schizophrenia in the sufferer. This raises two questions: what is the connection between brain chemistry and human thoughts and behaviour? And how can we fuse these two poles of explanation into some understanding of the human brain and its expression in the human being?

A CASE OF SCHIZOPHRENIA

Most people at some time or other have wondered how close they are to madness, but either have no way of finding out or shrink away from the opportunity. Richard Jameson grasped the nettle with both hands. He was an exceptionally bright young Oxford student who, in the summer of 1961, led the Oxford University Dramatic Society, as their President, on a tour of Northern Britain. In their adopted technique of 'method acting' the actor puts himself in the state of mind the character should be in. The key is for the actor to find the right feelings from within his own experience. Richard had to play a madman, and somewhere already within him a change had taken place, because he was indeed able to find the appropriate feelings. But he was all too successful; he really did go mad. He was admitted to hospital, and was diagnosed schizophrenic. What was the manifestation of his illness? Another of the student company, Esther Rantzen, now a familiar face on the TV screen, was deeply affected by what she witnessed:

> It's the only time I've ever seen a brilliant, as they say,
> normal young man go mad. It was completely formative.
> I now don't think of mental illness as something that
> happens to mad people. I think of it as something that
> could happen to any of us.

I can remember a tremendous physical change in him, that he became very gaunt, very taut, flushed as if he had a fever and in fact that remained a very lasting memory with me and it's made *me* believe there is a physical change with mental illness, that it *is* an illness. If you'd seen him, you'd have thought 'this is a man with a very high fever'.

How it affected him mentally was that he was talking perfectly coherently, except you didn't know what the heck he was on about. The only person who could relate to him in any way was a girl in the company . . . and she seemed to be able to follow his conversation, which took, say, strange kinds of spiritual leaps. He was talking in another realm, and every time you tried to respond to a sentence, you'd be terrified that it was the wrong response. . . .

THE SYMPTOMS OF THE PSYCHOSIS

Schizophrenia has defied simple definition ever since its conception by a Swiss psychiatrist, Eugen Bleuler, in 1911. It is a range of diseases and in the form that is recognized by its development in younger adults, the classic symptoms are bizarre. The sufferer has hallucinations and delusions. He often hears strange voices, conveying offensive messages, may become wild and irrational, and may sometimes become extremely withdrawn and unresponsive.

The form Richard developed was wild, ebullient; expressive on the surface, though very reticent when it came to his real emotional concerns. He certainly had crazy thinking – the crucial symptom – although he did not display the other common symptom of withdrawal and absence of reaction.

The medical controversy over the diseases called schizo-phrenia arises from the complexities and merging of these two different types of symptoms and their variants, continuing uncertainty about their causes and, of course, their diagnosis and their treatment.

Some psychiatrists believe schizophrenia is brought on by family pressures, but whether this was so in Richard's case we shall never know. Richard was very bright; he won scholarships successively to Winchester Cathedral choir, to Winchester College and to Magdalen College, Oxford. His father died when Richard was sixteen, his mother later remarried and moved out to Kenya, and all seemed well enough, until the events of 1961, and the ill-fated tour of the Dramatic Society.

It was at that point that Richard Jameson's life crumbled. Since then the pattern of his life has been a series of admissions, not always willing, to the corridors of mental hospitals. For years he lived in public wards, with scant attention, institutional food,

RICHARD'S YOUTH

Richard Jameson began life with excellent prospects. He excelled at prep school (he is shown on the far left) and won scholarships to Winchester School and Magdalen College, Oxford. Before his first breakdown Richard Jameson was not only President of the Oxford University Experimental Theatre Club (the ETC) but, as this review shows, was one of their best actors. His breakdown came when he was 22 while acting the part of a madman in a play at the Edinburgh Festival.

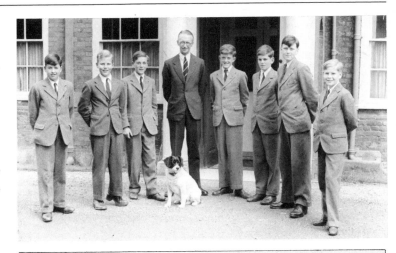

A 'certain success' for the E.T.C.

SIX curtain-calls. An Eights Week romp. Determined gaiety. Tinkling tunes. Pretty scenery. Delightful costumes. A sense of style. A turn for the better. A certain success? Undoubtedly.

A few reservations? Lack of projection. Ragged in places. Singing weak. Needs more polish. Needs more zip Needs more punch. Undoubtedly, too.

But the great virtue of the University Experimental Theatre Club musical at the Playhouse this week is that it is unpretentious in spirit and wonderfully light-hearted in effect.

Giles Havergal has produced an undergraduate vaudeville version of Labiche and Michel's 19th century French comedy, **An Italian Straw Hat,**

THEATRE

that tinkles along with infectious levity, that is as skittish as the plot of the play itself.

Adrian Brine's translation is witty (as probably are his lyrics if only the cast would sing loudly and clearly enough for us to hear them properly). Gordon Crosse's music, if slender and lacking in variety, is spirited and melodious and firmly played by the band of ten.

A delight

The scenery and costumes are a delight. John Marsh's simple, skeletal setting, enriched with lovely dresses by Auriol Stevens, stylish bric-a-brac and good lighting, serves this episodic chase across Paris after a hat admirably: enables the perpetual pursuit of the

wedding-party after our compromised bridegroom to proceed fluidly across the stage.

And the actors take their chances. Richard Jameson, as the man who spends his wedding-day saving a lady's honour, gives a particularly fine performance: easy, smooth, unruffled (perhaps at times a little too unruffled), but beautifully timed and the lines where necessary—such as: "I was only saying to myself this morning, 'What on earth shall I do this evening?'"—effortlessly thrown away.

John Wells scores a well-earned triumph as Tardiveau. David Robson, as Achille—"the orchid"—rounds off a delightful piece of foolery with one of the best presented songs of the evening. Romola Christopherson, as the Baroness, shares a charming number I-ta-lee, with Mr. Jameson. David Senton repeats his dapper lieutenant.

But, as is probably a tribute to the producer, all the characters are nicely etched—from the bride (Caroleen McFarlane) to the deaf uncle (Jeremy Bloggs)—and there are 24 of them.

The debits

What of the debits? Well, none of the songs end. They all stop suddenly. The bad vocal control of the singers makes most of them seem jerky. The need for a bit more projection and co-ordination shows up badly in the crowd scenes. Individual voices are often lost in the noise. The whole thing, one feels needs screwing up that bit tighter

We need a tidier can-can finale. An even more electric first-half curtain from Nicholas Mott (the tenor who can sing

But it is good. And I'll eat my straw hat if most people don't like it

DON CHAPMAN.

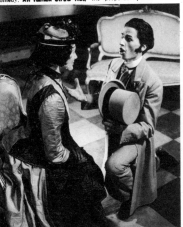

Richard Jameson, the hero of the Oxford University Experimental Theatre Club production of An Italian Straw Hat at the Playhouse, attempts a hurried explanation to Norma Rowan, the hat shop owner he has left in the lurch on his wedding day.

boredom and despair. Inside Richard's head there really was another world. His eyes and brain would see the same sights as the rest of us, but interpreted them with a logic of fantasy. It was not unlike the example of the schizophrenic who claimed to be the King of Poland and, when challenged, would show the label on his dressing gown and say, 'There's the proof.' The label would certainly read 'Made in Poland'. Richard's reactions were similar: when he believed he was God, an acquaintance said, 'What lousy weather we're having,' and Richard replied, 'Well, I'm doing my best!' What was being mad like for him?

> It is being out of control, not necessarily depressed or elated but in a dream world and unable to get through to anybody else who thinks you're mad. . . . Yes, I was mad and what a terrible situation I was in. It was like being clothed with a strait-jacket almost automatically. I realized that nothing I could say or do at that moment would alter the fact . . . they were quite right in saying that I was mad. There I was talking to them. . . . But I was mad and they weren't.

A FANTASY WORLD

Such insight was probably rare; for a lot of the time Richard's fantasies took over completely. Some of the disorders in his brain which led him to these exciting mind adventures can be analysed. Take this one for example.

> My mother was in league with the Queen to dupe the public into buying things like calendars and watches – there's no such thing as time. She started Richard Shops

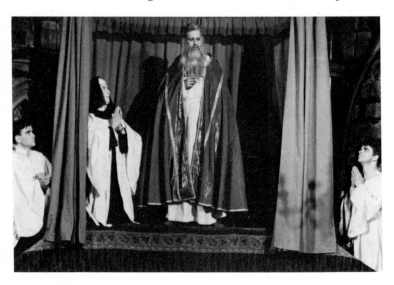

INTIMATIONS OF DIVINITY
Richard Jameson's memories of acting grand parts in productions such as *The World's Great Theatre* returned during his madness. 'I knew what it felt like to be God as I'd acted the part in a play.'

for me. And she had various crimes on her plate and I imagined a courtroom scene above my flat. I could hear every word of this trial and the buzz of the electrodes as they tortured my mother. And there was a BBC matron sort of type who was in charge of the court and she said, 'Do you want to say anything, Richard?' And I said, 'Yes, I do,' and I said this and that and the other and then she relayed it back to the Court because they couldn't hear. She said, 'Richard says such and such a thing,' and then my mother made some sort of garbled comment and it went on, I should say, for about half an hour. And my mother's tongue was cut out and she came down the steps screaming and yelling with her tongue cut out and was taken off to prison or something like that. Oh no, she didn't go to prison, she went to build her own walled garden. Most people were tortured or killed but she had the privilege of building her own walled garden from the inside, you see, so you eventually wall yourself in. Quite painless until you die of starvation in the end.

Hearing voices, and in this case also the buzz of electrodes, is a typical 'auditory hallucination', one of the more evident surface symptoms of schizophrenia. The second characteristic feature of this example was that Richard's thinking was disordered: about his mother, time, crime and so on. The two, disordered thinking and auditory hallucinations, combine together to give this strange waking dream. Crazy thinking obviously only takes place frequently in those who are mentally ill, but hallucinations, either of sounds or sights, can occur in normal people.

This experience of Richard's is similar to the kind of specific hallucination which other people suffer yet choose not to disclose. Many schizophrenics have such experiences over a number of years and remain undiscovered, undiagnosed, even carrying on with their normal work until they become overtly schizophrenic.

Richard's illness began to go further, and as well as producing isolated strange interludes, began to perpetrate an overall delusion concerning his place in the world. Indeed, his whole life became a fantasy.

I was the star of a huge film that was being made all over London with hidden cameras and microphones. And I found myself sitting in a café somewhere and talking to the hidden microphones, until the proprietor slung me out. It was marvellous when I went to Queensway Ice Rink and went on the ice and there were camera bulbs popping away and I thought, 'Oh, this is terrific, they're doing the whole thing,' and in fact it was one of those automatic photographic machines, you know, doing its popping away. But everything fitted into my dream and I was on cloud number nine.

This global delusion of Richard's shows that he was able to take real events in the outside world (the flash of the photo machine) and fit them into his crazy thought patterns. Here, the parts of his brain which deal with perception of sights, sounds, and other inputs from the senses were probably working normally; it was the interpretation in his head which was wrong.

ARE THERE ANY EXPLANATIONS?

As far as hallucinations are concerned, we can attempt to relate the effects of hypnosis with the standard techniques for observing changes in the brain to explain some of the symptoms of Richard's madness.

Consider the recorded instances of hypnosis in which the subjects are persuaded into visual hallucination. Not only have they been made to believe they can see something which does not exist, and describe it, but in other demonstrations they have accepted suggestions that they were blind.

In such circumstances the implication is that the subject still receives signals in the brain from his eyes, that the signals go through the brain's normal process for vision, but that the subject just refuses to admit that he can see. Tests have shown that, when the electrical activity of the appropriate region of the subject's brain is monitored, the result for the best of subjects has indicated no activity. The evidence of the EEG was that, as a result of hypnotic suggestion, the subject was able to switch off the visual cortex of his brain, to render himself 'blind'.

These results may be extended to apply to Richard Jameson's auditory hallucinations. If the brain, on which all our perceptions depend, can switch itself on and off, then in terms of brain activity his hallucinatory sounds – a switching on – could well be as real as any true sounds. That is how they seemed to him.

But what about Richard's fantasizing, for example, to the flash of the photo machine? The photo flash was a trivial event, which most people would ignore or filter out of their thoughts. He overreacted. Could it not be that the cells in some parts of his brain were over-sensitive to stimuli, and 'fired' in much greater numbers than in normal people, swamping the system and causing him eventually to lose his sense of reality?

This notion of abnormality in Richard's brain cells is supported by a strange scientific detective story which, more importantly, explains why Richard is back at work and not, as he puts it, 'locked up with a load of loonies'. We shall discover how there came to be a treatment for his disease.

DRUGS TO TREAT MADNESS

Before the 1950s there was no effective treatment for schizophrenia. The hospitals could sedate patients, but they often became completely inactive vegetables; alternatively, there was a range of questionable treatments for schizophrenia. Electro convulsive therapy, often known by its abbreviation ECT, was one of them; it involves passing an electric shock through the brain, and while it is still used for treating depression, on schizophrenia it had little effect. Several other treatments were used, among them injections of insulin, which resulted in the coma characteristic of diabetes; the powerful insulin hormone makes the body use up too much of its available sugar, the brain starves and the patient becomes unconscious. Treatment was crude, to say the least, and an effective alternative did not even seem to be in sight. It might not be even now, except for a happy accident.

In 1950 a French Navy surgeon, Henri Laborit, was working on methods for treating surgical shock, and for reducing the amounts of anaesthetic needed to keep his patients unconscious. He tested a range of drugs made by the company Rhone-Poulenc, with some success: the drugs seemed to reduce the shock that patients often show after operations using general anaesthetics. This prompted Rhone-Poulenc to make more chemicals and one of them, '4560 RP', was the best of the lot. Its soothing effects were so marked that other doctors were tempted to try it. In 1951 the control of new or experimental drugs by government was so loose that they could be given almost at the whim of a doctor to a guinea-pig patient and in this particular case that was a good thing: 4560 RP was an effective tranquillizer and within months it was being given to mentally ill patients. To everyone's surprise it had an effect on schizophrenia. This modest beginning heralded a revolution in the mental hospitals. Sales of the drug rocketed.

HOSPITAL POPULATION AND DRUGS

The anti-schizophrenic drugs, or 'major tranquillizers' such as Largactil and Modecate, were first used in the 1960s. They controlled the symptoms of schizophrenia so successfully that the mental hospital population was rapidly reduced. But these drugs do not cure, and many schizophrenics are re-admitted to hospital.

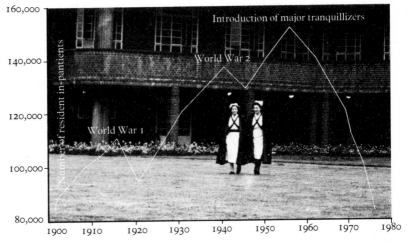

And the hospitals opened their doors. Previously uncontroll-able schizophrenic or manic patients were now easy to handle, were much less likely to harm themselves, or others, or behave in a socially unacceptable way. There were clearly two factors in this revolution: the drug reduced some of the worst symptoms of the disease; but it also made the patients easier for the institutions and society to handle and accept. These phenothiazines, or anti-schizophrenic drugs as they came to be called, are as useful to the institutions as to the patients. But perhaps one should neither be surprised nor condemnatory about that: it did lead to the release of tens of thousands of patients from the caring prisons we call mental hospitals, even if that freedom brought inevitable practical problems.

The drugs were not discovered by scientists searching for a treatment for schizophrenia, but by a series of fortunate intuitions leading from the operating table to the locked mental ward. They alleviated the symptoms. A soothing effect is one part of the drugs' action: they also make certain schizophrenics think more clearly and coherently. They do not work in all schizophrenics and they do not cure, they merely hold the worst symptoms, the thought disorders, in check. Patients still get hallucinations and delusions, though they are reduced. Obviously, they are less intrusive anyway once the patient begins to think more coherently. But if we could find out just why the drugs do work, that should lead to better drugs in the future; and to some chance of understanding the disease and its causes.

THE HUNT FOR CLUES

Richard Jameson benefits from taking such a drug. 'It just takes the rough edges off your frame, off your existence.' But one side-effect of these drugs, which many – including Richard – experience is a severe, uncontrollable shaking of the limbs. Doctors noticed immediately that it resembled one of the classic symptoms of Parkinson's Disease (discussed in detail in the chapter on movement). Why should a drug that controls madness mimic the 'shaking palsy', a disease which seems to be entirely physical? Was there a connection between Parkinson's Disease and schizophrenia?

The first clue was that the symptoms of Parkinson's Disease could be relieved (but not cured) by a simple drug called L-DOPA. Unlike the anti-schizophrenic phenothiazine drugs, it is a natural constituent of body and brain. In the body L-DOPA is made into dopamine, one of the several neuro-transmitters, the chemicals which carry signals from one nerve end to another across the synapse. Dopamine is used by nerves throughout the body, but specifically in some nerve cells in the brain, significantly in a region in the brain that controls movement. Parkinson's Disease patients suffer because of a lack of dopamine, and when L-DOPA is given to

A DRUG COCKTAIL
Below is shown Richard Jameson's regular drug intake to control the symptoms of schizophrenia.

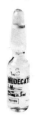

Modecate: A monthly injection which diffuses slowly into his bloodstream and controls the symptoms of schizophrenia.

Largactil: The first of the anti-schizophrenic drugs to be developed, which is more tranquillizing than Modecate.

Haloperidol (Serenace): A later and more effective anti-schizophrenic drug which 'tops up' the Modecate injection.

Disipal: Partially counteracts the side effects of the three anti-schizophrenic drugs, such as severe trembling of his limbs.

Lithium (Priadel): This controls Richard's second condition: swings of mood from very 'high' to very depressed.

them it is turned to dopamine in movement regions of the brain that lack it. Were the anti-schizophrenic drugs depleting dopamine in the brain, including those movement areas, so causing Parkinsonian tremor?

Such questions led to the theory that schizophrenia was caused by an overactive dopamine system (the reverse of the case in Parkinson's Disease) in which a small stimulus, such as Richard's photo flash at the ice-rink, could cause many more nerves to fire than normal because there was more neuro-transmitter to pass signals from one nerve to the next. The general result would be a brain that reacted in a wild, illogical way and was oversensitive to every sort of stimulus, including emotional ones, showing marked symptoms of schizophrenia.

TESTING A THEORY

Since Largactil, as the original drug is called, obviously does interfere with movements controlled by the brain's dopamine, it was worth studying that connection in detail in case it was related to the drug's anti-schizophrenic activity, rather than merely to the unwanted side-effects on movement. To many scientists that seemed simple enough. The effect of Largactil on other types of nerves was tested, and it was shown that Largactil affected virtually every nerve cell in the brain and body, even those controlling the use of oxygen in each breath we take. But the tests were not specific enough to establish precisely what the drug's effect really is on schizophrenia.

It was a Swedish scientist, Arvid Carlsson, who made the next advance. Carlsson first checked to see if Largactil affected the rate at which a rat made and then eventually broke down dopamine. He reasoned that the drug might be blocking the places where dopamine normally acted, that is the receptor sites, thereby slowing down the dopamine nerves' activity. The nerve cells would sense this, and 'assume' that it was because they were not making enough dopamine. So they would make more to try and counteract the drug's effect. And once there was more dopamine around, it would automatically be broken down faster. But why should the effect on dopamine be relevant to schizophrenia?

Carlsson knew that Largactil affected lots of other body chemicals. He reasoned that if dopamine was connected with schizophrenia, then the more active a drug in relieving the symptoms of schizophrenia, the more effect it should have on dopamine. By that time several other drugs had been developed and one of them, haloperidol, was a hundred times more effective against schizophrenia than Largactil. Carlsson showed that haloperidol also had a greater effect on the rat's manufacture and break-down of dopamine. What is more, a drug chemically similar to Largactil, but with no anti-schizophrenic activity, did not increase the rat's turnover of dopamine. It was the first direct connection between the anti-schizophrenic drugs and dopamine; between madness and the brain's chemistry. Carlsson's theory was that the drugs, both dopamine and the anti-schizophrenic drugs, fitted into receptor sites on the nerve cells, like keys fitting into locks. It was some years, however, before a technique was developed (in the USA) to test the theory.

Scientists in America took the anti-schizophrenic drugs and made them radio-active, so that even a tiny amount could be detected wherever it was. They took from a rat's brain nerve cells that use dopamine, and added the radio-active drug to them. It stuck to the nerve cells' synapses, one of Carlsson's predictions. In theory, the drug would prevent the dopamine from sticking, and so from passing signals from one nerve to the next. So far the evidence was inconclusive, however, because there was no way of knowing if the radio-active drugs were occupying the sites normally reserved by dopamine, thereby displacing it. To solve this location riddle they added dopamine at the same time as the radio-active drug. If both stuck to the same receptors, they would compete with each other and radio-active count would be lower. Sure enough, less radio-activity stuck to the nerves when dopamine was present as well. The little lock into which the dopamine 'key' fitted was just the right shape for the drug key as well.

When Richard Jameson takes his daily cocktail of drugs, which includes both Largactil and haloperidol, they make their way into his bloodstream, cross the blood-brain barrier, find their way to the synapses of the dopamine nerve cells in his brain, and stick there. Then, when a nerve signal passes from one such cell, in the presence of the drugs it has to be a much stronger signal than normal to activate an adjoining cell. The dopamine released by the first cell cannot all stick to the second cell since many of its receptors are already occupied by drug molecules.

DOPAMINE LEVELS IN THE BRAIN

These were the results for nerve cells from a rat's brain. How could the dopamine theory be proved in human beings? Dopamine could not be measured in living brains, for obvious reasons, so Cambridge University embarked on the long-term and somewhat macabre project of collecting brains from dead schizophrenic patients. They now have hundreds, deep-frozen, potentially one of the most valuable collections of biological material in the world. Each brain was sliced and the dopamine-rich areas carefully cut out in a project involving Dr Leslie Iversen, and now Dr Martin Rosser and their collaborators. They found that there was indeed more dopamine in the schizophrenic brains than in normal brains. But there was still a problem. Nearly all schizophrenics in Britain take the anti-schizophrenic drugs, and so did the patients whose brains Iversen

THE NERVE JUNCTION
A) Within the brain are billions of junctions like this between adjacent nerve cells.
B) One type uses a simple chemical, dopamine, which transfers signals across the junction, or synapse, by fitting into receptors in the second cell. In schizophrenia there may be a disorder of this mechanism causing the second cell to fire too often.
C) This is held in check by the anti-schizophrenic drugs which block receptors and reduce the response of the second cell and likewise, cells all over the dopamine regions of the brain.

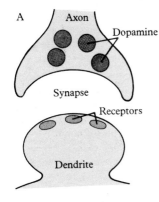

A · Axon · Dopamine · Synapse · Receptors · Dendrite

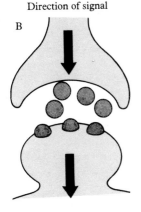

Direction of signal

B

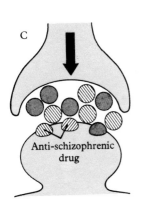

C

Anti-schizophrenic drug

and Rosser examined. So why did they contain so much dopamine, which should have been suppressed by the drug?

Remember that when a patient first takes the drugs, they block the dopamine receptors. So the cell is receiving less dopamine than before. The cell seems to be able to detect the difference between dopamine and the drugs, even though both fit into the same places. It therefore sends out a message (undoubtedly a special chemical) which informs other cells, 'I'm not receiving as much dopamine as usual.' The other cells respond by making more dopamine, and that process continues. When the patient dies, there will be more dopamine than usual in the brain. A similar 'feed-back' mechanism causes an increase in the number of dopamine receptors, so the whole dopamine system is enlarged.

So, while we now have a better understanding of the activity of the anti-schizophrenic drugs via the dopamine system, we are much less sure about the precise nature of the connection between dopamine and schizophrenia. Dopamine does seem to increase by about a fifth in schizophrenics who have never taken drugs, but that increase is not enough to enable Drs Leslie Iversen and Tim Crow and their colleagues, the British scientists doing this work, to conclude that schizophrenia is caused primarily by damage to the dopamine system. No wonder the drugs do not cure it: but they leave us with the question as to why they alleviate the symptoms.

THE DRUG SCENE

In Britain, Dr Sue Iversen, Dr Leslie Iversen's wife, has been using amphetamine in the study of schizophrenia. (For some time it has been known that amphetamine, taken over a long period of time, will – in human beings – mimic the symptoms of schizophrenia.) She believes that the involvement of dopamine in the disease is more complex than was at first thought. She suggests three different dopamine systems. When amphetamine is fed to animals such as rats or monkeys it affects all the three dopamine systems they have in their brains. They become very agitated, and also repeat various movements for hours on end. Such movements are particular to each species, and become more complicated the closer the animal is to man: rats gnaw, cats groom and scratch. These movements are controlled by one of the three dopamine systems: this one is part of the brain system which causes the trembling side-effects. In schizophrenic humans, these symptoms, according to Sue Iversen, are also repetitive, but much more sophisticated than in animals. Schizophrenics will empty and refill handbags, or endlessly polish furniture or, as Richard did in the early stages of his first attack, throw cup after British Rail cup out of a train window. Schizophrenic clockmakers will endlessly build and dismantle bits of their clocks; mechanics will do the same with cars.

The second dopamine system in the brain, Dr Iversen believes, is connected with hallucinations and delusions. It is in the frontal part of the cerebral hemispheres. If a rat has this pathway removed by the injection of a poisonous drug and is then put into a new laboratory cage with food, water and so on, it will apathetically sit and do nothing. A normal rat would soon explore to find out what is there. A rat dosed with amphetamine and thus mimicking schizophrenia, would, like a human schizophrenic, over-explore. It would not know which object to take seriously, would be over-reactive to many of them (as Richard was to the photo flash) and may even begin to react to objects which don't exist (like Richard's voices). In general the amphetamine rat or schizophrenic human is over-aroused.

The third dopamine system controls response to stress: schizophrenics do over-react to stress of any sort, especially emotional stress, and the third dopamine system may be the part of the brain involved in this, but the evidence is vague and uncertain.

The one key symptom of schizophrenia not covered by these animal studies is disordered thinking. That may merely reflect how difficult it is to find out what animals *are* thinking! It may also point towards the true primary cause of schizophrenia: a chemical error outside the dopamine system, though still in the brain.

A REFINED THEORY

Arvid Carlsson was also an early investigator of the effects of the psychedelic drugs. His original interest in drugs and the brain has been fertile. Scattered around Sweden are his ex-students, now making Sweden a centre for research into brain chemistry. One of them, Professor Urban Ungerstedt, has alternatives to the dopamine hypothesis. He is studying the chemistry of the brains of living animals. This is a major new method because until now scientists have only been able to monitor the *electrical activity* of brain cells, whereas signals are transferred from cell to cell by chemical means. It has taken ten years to develop the technique, really an artificial blood vessel inside the rat's brain. Ungerstedt's colleagues insert into the brain a plastic tube a mere one hundredth of an inch thick, which can either be used to feed the brain with drugs, or to collect minute samples of the brain's secretions for analysis. Professor Ungerstedt gives rats amphetamine to mimic human schizophrenia, and then measures the change in dopamine and other neuro-transmitters in the fluid slowly dripping out from the tube. Dopamine does change, but so do two other chemicals that the techniques are sensitive enough to detect, glutamic acid and GABA (Gamma Amino Butyric Acid), both of which are recently-discovered neuro-transmitters. The former works in cells which connect up with the dopamine cells. From this and related evidence Professor Ungerstedt and other scientists now believe that the

NEUROTIC OR PSYCHOTIC? These two paintings, widely differing in period and style, present powerful images of two of the major forms of mental disorder. Romantic artists, such as the Swiss painter, Johann Heinrich Fuseli (1741-1825), were fascinated by the often bizarre workings of the human mind. In *Mad Kate* Fuseli exploits the layers of horror, fear and elation in his subject's disordered brain (*top*). In contrast, the 20th-century American painter George Tooker depicts the isolation, stress and fear of the neurotic in *The Subway* (1950).

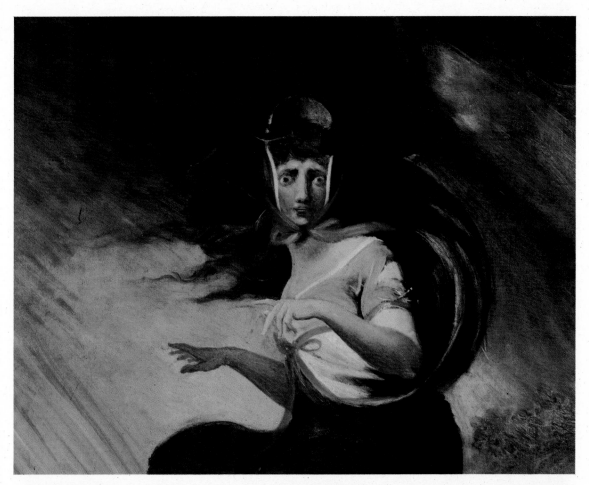

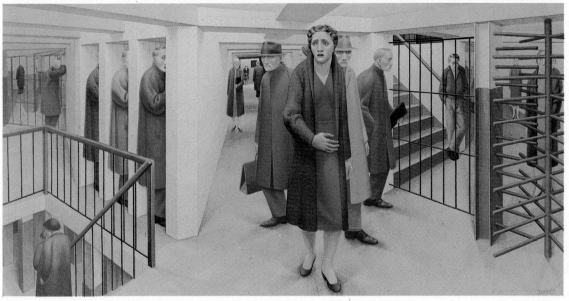

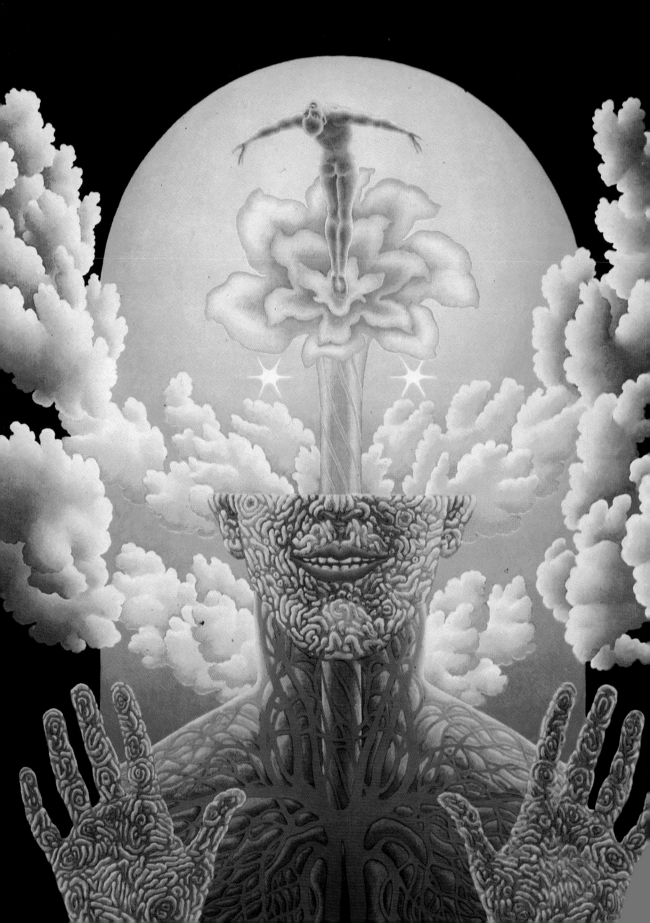

TWO INTO ONE WON'T GO
The belief in an entity called the mind, which is independent of the human brain is common to many cultures. This illustration, painted by Justin Todd for a book entitled, *Centre of the Cyclone*, is one expression of this dualistic idea. Many scientists and philosophers are monists who believe that we are nothing more than the workings of our brain (*see page 163*).

primary fault which causes madness is not in the dopamine system, but some other type of brain cell that connects with it. They are testing drugs in cells that use glutamic acid and hope that this will lead to a more effective treatment for Richard and other schizophrenics. But even if their theories turn out to be correct, development of a drug for human use will take years, or even decades.

CONFRONTING THE REAL WORLD

Schizophrenia is clearly related to chemical disorder in the brain, but this does not mean that a person's environment, social or otherwise, is unimportant. Relatives, friends and surroundings could well precipitate the illness, or alternatively keep it in check, and they can undoubtedly be a major factor in recovery. Richard spent several periods in hospitals that were poorly run, and can tell of experiences and regimes that would have undermined the most stable personality. Vicious nurses (not a common occurrence, thankfully); hospitals of one or two thousand disturbed inmates; queues to see doctors; none of this is remotely conducive to recovery.

He was fortunate that, at his tenth admission, he encountered sympathy and caring in a smaller hospital, with a small psychiatric unit. In that more protective environment, a smaller establishment run as a therapeutic community with an emphasis on social interaction, Richard – still helped by his drugs – began to experience a form of recuperation. And there did come the day when he was considered fit for discharge. Now, twenty years after the first attack, is he cured?

> It's been a matter of bouts, you know, bouts for various reasons, interspersed by say a couple of years or five years of perfect health. I've just been out of hospital for five or six years and I'm just due for my next bout. I hope it doesn't happen. I very much hope it doesn't happen because I'm making desperately sure that I'm all right all the time.

We still do not know exactly what caused Richard's illness. But because of the discovery of new drugs, and sympathetic hospital treatment, he is able to lead a useful life, where thirty years ago he would have been confined to an institution. Investigations into the brain's chemical mysteries will continue, and eventually we shall know the chemical basis of madness.

CHAPTER 7

THE SELF: CONSCIOUSNESS

Imagine, for a moment, that it is possible to remove your brain from your skull, but to keep it in contact with the rest of your body by some sort of radio-link. Both your brain and your body, as long as the radio communication is in operation, function as they do in their more usual arrangement. Your brain, for the sake of illustration, is kept functioning in a vat of fluid, and a life-support system will see that its temperature and so forth are as they should be. Now imagine that you, that is to say all the parts of you except your brain, are looking at this isolated brain, removed from your skull, floating in its glass chamber. Where would *you* be? Hidden behind the glass, or staring through the glass at three and a half pounds of fatty tissue?

WHERE IS YOUR SELF?

It's difficult not to feel that you, yourself – your *self* – would be the body looking at the brain. Somehow, it would be difficult to take one's brain, in those circumstances, much more seriously than the appendix which a surgeon might keep floating in a jar of formaldehyde. Not many people, of course, would believe that the elusive self, or mind, or consciousness, was located in the appendix, any more than in the left foot, or even in the heart. There is not much doubt nowadays that *if it has any material location* it must be in the brain.

All of us feel that we possess a unique individuality, and that individuality we describe variously, using such imprecise and non-technical terms as mind, self (our choice for this chapter), soul, spirit, and the like.

We have all heard the phrase, 'Not enough to keep body and soul together'. That particular saying conveys something of the common man's view of himself, that as a human being he is made up of two parts, the physical body which is controlled by the brain, and a second, non-physical component which constitutes some overall power, the 'soul' in the terms of our example, indivisible from and integral to the body.

In this chapter on the self we seek to explore the part, if any, which the brain might play in understanding or controlling itself. We shall consider alternative theories in the brain/mind debate, and by comparing the way in which damaged brains operate with the way in which normal brains operate we can attempt to throw light on the functioning of the normal brain.

MONISTS AND DUALISTS

Monism, or materialism, is the belief that the mind does not exist separately from the brain. Dualism is the belief that it does. There are shades of opinion between these extremes, and many brain scientists do not believe wholeheartedly in monism, though it is probably fair to say that the majority reject the doctrine of dualism. Not all materialists are students of the biology of the brain. A philosopher, who is also a materialist, is Professor Daniel Dennett, from Tufts University, Boston. Dennett:

> What the dualist does, inspired by the quite correct intuition that you can't just locate the self like a little nugget somewhere in the brain – what the dualist does is invent a magical space and inhabit it with some new substance, the mind, as if that solved the problem. But that couldn't solve the problem – that is just giving up. It leaves all the truly interesting questions of how the mind

WHERE AM I?
Professor Daniel Dennett viewing a 'working model' of his own brain and pondering the location of his self. 'Why do I feel as if I'm out here looking at my own brain, rather than in the being viewed by my own body?'

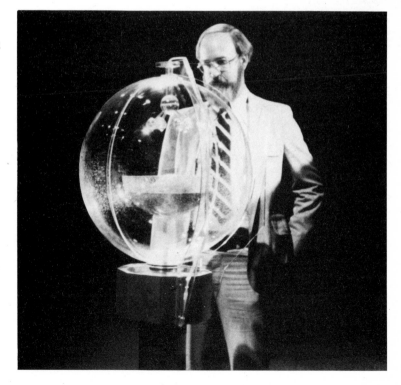

works, not only unanswered, but unanswerable. No
dualist has yet proposed any tests or devices for
measuring the activity of the non-physical mind, and in
fact if one were to propose such a test, I think the dualists
would say, 'Well, whatever you are testing, it can't be
the non-physical mind, because that is in principle
beyond the ken of science.' But once that card has been
played, we can see that the dualist is really advocating a
council of despair and saying: 'There are these mysteries
and we cannot address them, so we can cover our
embarrassment by inventing a mysterious substance
called the mind, and sweeping all the difficult problems
under that spectral rug.'

It would be difficult to find any more distinguished brain scientist
than Sir John Eccles, who is a dualist. He believes that the mind and
the brain are separate entities, and so he is unable to suggest any
material substance of which the mind might be composed. Sir John
Eccles was a pupil of the pioneer of modern neuro-science, Sir
Charles Sherrington, as far back as the late 1920s (see Chapter 4 on
movement). When he left Sherrington's laboratories in Oxford he
carved out a most substantial career on the frontiers of brain
physiology. Brilliant, charming, energetic, dogmatic and at times
alarming, Eccles is now almost eighty. He still attends many
international conferences at which he makes his views heard, and
sometimes felt. His views about the hemispheres of the brain are
characteristically straightforward.

I don't think it [*the right hemisphere*] is a conscious self. I
don't think it worries about tomorrow, I don't think it
worries about, shall we say, moral problems about what
it should do, and so on. I think that kind of thing,
altruistic behaviour and so forth, are entirely left
hemisphere functions, going with self-consciousness.
But the right hemisphere has consciousness of a more
sophisticated kind that we have been able to show even
in chimpanzees. So that is the answer. You haven't split
the soul, the psyche, into two. You have in the right
hemisphere some kind of primitive concept of self, but
not a real self-consciousness associated with the human
psyche or the human person. I think the word person is
important. I use the word person for a subject who is
responsible for his actions, and the left hemisphere is a
human person, or associated with a human person,
whereas the right hemisphere is not.

Sir John Eccles is at pains to point out that all input from the senses,
and even our thinking, involves the behaviour of nerve cells.

THE PAIN GATE

A potentially painful stimulus, here burns on the body, may travel as a message as far as the spinal cord where it can be controlled by a gate-type mechanism. As a result, little or no pain may be experienced. Within the brain there are further such gates.

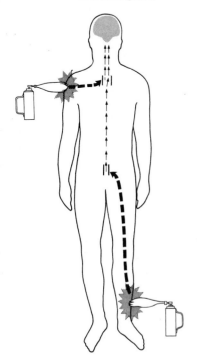

Since he himself established many of the connections between the actions of nerve cells and animal behaviour, it is a position he could certainly be expected to take. He believes that sensory impressions, though they are relayed to the brain by nerve signals, are subject to the interpretation of the mind. He cites the example of pain:

'You may get a lot of nerve cells firing in the brain, and you feel a pain. But there is no pain in the world at all. It is you who have made the pain. And the pain isn't explained by all this firing of cells, it is read out by you and you suffer with it; but you created your own pains.'

THE PROBLEM OF PAIN

We shall take Sir John's cue, and pursue the example of pain, a subject which has absorbed a number of students of consciousness. Historically, one of the most important pieces of research was that done by an army doctor, H K Beecher, on the beach-heads at Anzio. Beecher found that many men with very severe injuries felt, or at least reported, very little severe pain. Beecher decided that the subjective feeling of pain appeared to be regulated to a much larger degree than expected by the mental state of the injured man. It is certainly a common experience that accidents during, say, an energetic game of football, are not noticed until after the game. Pain, therefore, can to some degree be regarded as a subjective phenomenon. But that is not necessarily to say that there is no physical cause for such a subjective feeling. One proposed mechanism for which there is biological evidence is that there is, as it were, a 'gate' in the spinal cord which decides how much of the pain message should be transmitted and to where it should be transmitted. Thus a set of nerve cells decides the subjective feeling of pain, allotting to any injury the appropriate amount of pain, depending, presumably, on the circumstances. The major proponent of this theory is Professor Patrick Wall, of University College, London.

Patrick Wall is an unashamed materialist, who is prepared to substantiate a hypothesis by experimenting on himself. Consider an experiment which was concerned not directly with his 'gate' theory of pain, but with his theory that pain, or the experience of it, is one part of a spectrum of behaviour. Like any other form of behaviour, it will provide physical evidence that can be observed. Accordingly, Professor Wall attached electrodes to himself to measure his heart-rate and his rate of breathing. Then he plunged his forearm into a deep tank of water and crushed ice. Even without the evidence of the oscilloscope, it was clear that Wall suffered severe pain. His heart rate increased and his rate of breathing increased. When the pain became unbearable, Wall withdrew his arm and his heart rate and respiration began to fall to normal levels. His interpretation of the experiment was as follows:

The classical view, really an intuitive view, is that pain or the observation of it is a two-stage process. First the body, mechanics, delivering a pure sensation: and then something quite separate, the mind, examining that pure sensation and deciding whether it is good, bad, whether you hate it and so forth. I find that separation to be an artificial one. It is a convenient one to think of, but one continually sees that, in a real situation, I am not speaking now of curious laboratory situations, pain comes as a package. As you feel it, you hate it, and at the same time there are these huge integrated changes of the entire body, and all this occurs simultaneously. Now people go further with this idea of separating first the body and then the mind, and actually attempt to locate the mind. I think that is a deep misunderstanding, because I believe that the mind is a process of the brain, and not something that can be extracted.

What does Wall mean by a process of the brain? He uses an analogy to illustrate his theory. If one imagines a normal brain's constituent parts, they are like the parts of a machine. The brain cells do not show pain, or for that matter love or hate or green or red. Thus far, Eccles would agree. If we consider what we ordinarily think of as a machine, a motor-bike, once again it has constituent parts. But when a motor-cycle is being driven on a racing circuit, we can see that it has also a quality we call speed – and other qualities, such as noise or danger. But no speed, noise, or danger are among the parts listed by the manufacturer, nor were they included when the machine was assembled. They have no material existence. But Wall argues that we can think of the properties of the brain in the same way: pain is produced by the brain, just as speed is produced by the motor-bike. It is not a thing, even an immaterial thing, but a process. The mind and the brain cannot be separated.

Wall believes, moreover, that pain is not only a signal of injury but a form of behaviour. He thinks of pain in the same way as he thinks of thirst or hunger, which are signals of a body's state but are also the onset of a form of behaviour. In the case of hunger, behaviour will be to search for food; in the case of pain, the behaviour will be to search for means to overcome the injury which has caused the pain – to rest or seek for relief. He extends this theory to purely intellectual activities.

Now, quite obviously there are aspects of the mind which are not concerned with overt behaviour. I may be sitting and thinking. But I believe that those aspects of the mind can be seen in the same context, but more as a rehearsal. What would happen if I did something, for the moment I'm not going to do anything, but I will rehearse the possibilities. This then puts even your conscious thinking, without behaviour, into the context of normal behaviour.

The implication is that all human thought, including beliefs, values and morals, can be related to physical activity, either in the real world or rehearsed in our internal world of the brain.

Wall is a biologist, so does he see man as merely an animal, and almost dismiss the unique capabilities of the human mind?

'I do not see us at all as simple machinery, and we are clearly different from animals. But to say we are like animals is not an insult at all to me. Animals are also marvellous creatures, and I think that to say man is just a simple mechanism is a total misunderstanding of what people like myself are saying. We are not saying that man is like a watch or like a clockwork mouse. A real mouse is as different from a clockwork mouse as I think man is from a simple mechanism.'

The Physical Brain and the Conscious Mind

Pain may originate with sensory impressions relayed to the brain by nerve signals, but eminent men like Sir John Eccles and Professor Patrick Wall are at odds over the role of the brain in relation to the 'mind' in what happens next. At this point, then, it is appropriate to look closer at the relation between the physical activities of the brain and the working of the conscious mind. We shall examine particularly the outcome of a certain kind of brain surgery.

Earlier in this chapter we considered the intriguing proposition of a brain separated from but still linked to its host body. We are, of course, a long way from being able to realize such an experiment. But there are situations in which the human brain and its representation of mind, consciousness, or self, can be examined as a consequence of physical changes (though they are less dramatic than our hypothetically detached brain). The most energetic discussion in recent years about the nature of consciousness derives from a series of brain surgery cases. They are usually referred to as the split-brain cases.

All the patients had suffered from epilepsy of a serious and intractable kind, in which the electrical disorders had spread from a focus in one part of the brain to affect the whole mass of brain, resulting in violent convulsions and subsequent severe physical damage, head injuries and so forth. It had been known since 1940 that some relief could be obtained in such cases by isolating the two hemispheres of the brain from one another, and this procedure was adopted by Joseph Bogen, a surgeon in Los Angeles. Later, other surgeons became interested, and a few have continued to perform the operation until the present day. The early operations cut the corpus callosum, the thick bundle of nerve fibres which connect the two halves of the cerebral cortex, and also divided some other brain structures, sometimes including part of the fornix and part of the thalamus. Later studies suggested that, since the operation was a very large one in any case, it would be sufficient to divide only the corpus callosum. The severity of the operation, even in its more limited form, has caused the medical team or teams concerned to limit its use very strictly. Only a few operations of this kind are performed each year, and prospective patients are screened with the utmost care to ensure that less drastic treatment cannot relieve symptoms which have become totally unacceptable at any level of existence.

The immediate effects of severing the 50 million nerve fibres of the corpus callosum are threefold: input from the senses which arrives in the left hemisphere of the brain will no longer be carried to the right, and vice versa; instructions from one hemisphere will no longer go directly to the other; and, rather gratifyingly, the patient quite often experiences considerable relief of his epilepsy. The surgical procedure is remarkable. But it is only afterwards that it is possible to see the astonishing results of the split-brain procedure on the mental processes of the patient. They shed a bizarre light on the many questions about our consciousness, mind, and self.

HEMISPHERES OF INFLUENCE

A great deal of nonsense has been spoken and written about the two halves of the brain. Fantasy and science fiction are unnecessary – the facts are clear. In essence, the left hemisphere of the brain controls much of the right side of the body, and the right side of the brain controls much of the left side of the body, some functions being controlled by either hemisphere. Thus the right hand, for example, is under the control of the left hemisphere. More

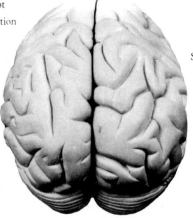

LEFT HEMISPHERE
CONTROLS

Right hand and foot

Arithmetic/calculation

Language

Right visual field

Smell from
right nostril

RIGHT HEMISPHERE
CONTROLS

Left hand and foot

Spatial perception

Left visual field

Smell from left nostril

LEFT AND RIGHT BRAINS
Generally the left hemisphere controls movements on the right side of the body and vice versa, but some movements, such as those of trunk, shoulders and hips are controlled by either side. Language is analyzed and produced by the left hemisphere in all but one person in 20, who are left-handers. In normal individuals the two hemispheres are in communication all the time, but if the connection between them is severed, bizarre effects of the split brain can be revealed by psychological tests.

remarkable, a discovery in the 1860s by the French scientist, Paul Broca, revealed that it is from the left half, the left hemisphere, of the brain that the ability to speak is nearly always controlled (see Chapter 2 on language). Indeed, the major capacity for language as a whole is found in the left hemisphere. It is this hemisphere that is normally dominant; it can suppress an attempt by the right hemisphere to communicate. But the right hemisphere controls certain skills which the left cannot, including spatial abilities such as drawing, map reading or finding one's way around. Popularly, the left hemisphere is identified with the analytical scientist and the right hemisphere with the creative artist, but the evidence for this is sparse and speculative. And, after all, both hemispheres are normally in contact, and in normal brains it only takes a couple of thousandths of a second for the 50 million nerve fibres to carry signals from one side to the other.

In the 1950s and early 1960s, Roger Sperry and Michael Gazzaniga had been conducting research at the California Institute of Technology on monkeys whose brains had been divided. As early as the 1940s the operation had been performed on humans in efforts to reduce the effects of epileptic seizures, and the patients did gain some relief but otherwise seemed to suffer no loss of physical performance as a result of their split brains. But Sperry and Gazzaniga's work in California showed that the corpus callosum, in particular, did carry information from one hemisphere to the other and enabled the brain to act as one unit, and that when the corpus callosum was divided the hemispheres seemed to become largely independent of each other. At the time they were conducting this animal research, there were no human patients available. When, therefore, it turned out that the split-brain, or commissurotomy, operation was being performed on humans by Bogen, Sperry and Gazzaniga approached him to see if any of his patients could be made available for testing.

TESTING A SPLIT BRAIN
The person being tested is shown a picture on the left for a split second, so that it is only perceived by his or her right hemisphere. In most cases that hemisphere cannot speak, and because of the patient's surgery cannot pass information to the left hemisphere. However, the right hemisphere controls the left hand and the subject can pick out the object correctly. The right hand cannot pick out the object as it neither saw the original picture, nor can it see the five choices due to the opaque screen.

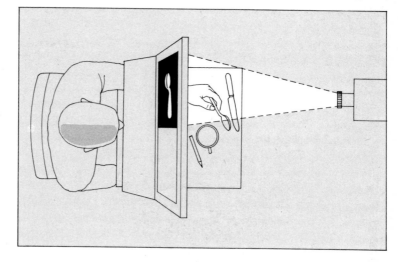

The curious thing about the patients, when Sperry and Gazzaniga first met them, was that there was nothing curious about them! Each hemisphere was receiving the same information from the environment at the same time, and in normal social conduct and conversation the patients appeared perfectly normal. Neurological examinations of the patients did show some differences in behaviour between their left and right hands though. Some patients were unable to name objects – pencils, paper clips, drawing pins – held in the left hand, which is controlled by the right hemisphere. But the most fascinating results came when Sperry and Gazzaniga began their psychological tests.

There seemed to be two separate streams of consciousness running through each patient. One stream was related to the left hemisphere, and the other to the right, and they seemed to have their own quite separate sensations and perceptions, even their own memories. There were even, apparently, two visual systems, in the sense that one system, the left, could see and talk about what it had seen, whereas the right or minor hemisphere, while it could see, was unable adequately to describe or comment on what it had seen. But there was a weird corollary to this observation. With their left hands, the subjects were able to point at the material which they had seen with their right hemispheres. But there seemed to be no communication between the two hemispheres. Were there two minds in one brain?

Roger Sperry for many years pursued a career of the greatest distinction in the brain sciences, culminating in the Nobel Prize in 1981. He is still at the California Institute of Technology and still interests himself in the commissurotomy cases from the early 1960s. He has continued to investigate and refine his experimental techniques in collaboration with colleagues. And, perhaps prompted by the strangeness of the split-brain cases, he has become fascinated with the problems and definitions of consciousness.

THE STORY OF VICKI

Roger Sperry's collaborator, Michael Gazzaniga, has gone east, to New York. His research work brings him into contact with split-brain patients from the Great Lakes area. Vicki is one such patient, who travels the 600 miles from her Ohio home to New York, where she confesses to enjoying Gazzaniga's tests.

She is an attractive, dark-haired woman in her early thirties, divorced, and with an eight-year-old daughter, Angel, who lives with her. Since her operation Vicki no longer has so many crippling *grand mal* epileptic seizures, although almost every day she will have a mild attack – a *petit mal*. Her life is scarcely plain sailing. When she came out of hospital, she stayed with her parents, who cared for Angel and looked for an apartment for Vicki. At last they found a run-down apartment, and her father and brother helped to get it ready. Vicki is unemployed, and does not drive because of her recurrent epileptic attacks. She is looking for voluntary work, because the two most obvious sources of employment are closed to her: she can't type and she can't be a waitress because her manual dexterity is limited through her operation. Vicki knows, too, and knew before she started her psychological tests, that there was a strangeness in her behaviour.

> My left hand is under control, but yet it grabs things that it shouldn't grab, or it grabs things I don't want it to grab. It just sort of just reaches out, like that. I don't like the idea of that, because I don't know what is happening. Sometimes I just take my right hand and grab hold of my left hand or arm and pull it back. Other times, it may sound silly, but I slap it because I get mad at it, I really do, I get really mad at it, and I find that doesn't do any good, except it hurts after it's slapped.

Typical of this behaviour are the repeated frustrations she experiences when trying to select her clothes in the morning. 'I knew what I wanted to wear and I would open my closet, get ready to take out what I wanted, and my other hand would just take control. It would just reach in. I told the lady at medical college that I was really fighting with it and she said to talk to it, talk to your hand. But it didn't do any good. It would reach in and get something I didn't want at all. And a couple of times I had a pair of shorts on, and I would find myself putting on another pair of shorts on top of the pair I already had on. I knew that was wrong. I wouldn't go out of the house that way, I knew that was totally wrong, but my hand sort of took control, got that other pair of shorts and put them on.'

The rogue hand, of course, is her left one. Is there a right Vicki as well as a left Vicki? And have her mind and her self split, as the surgeon split the two hemispheres of her brain?

DEFINING TWO SELVES

The purpose of Michael Gazzaniga's tests is to establish exactly what is going on inside Vicki's head. In the laboratory where Gazzaniga works with Vicki and one assistant, he tries to keep the atmosphere intimate and friendly. But the light-hearted atmosphere cannot disguise the profundity of the questions which his apparently simple tests are asking.

For the tests, Gazzaniga uses a translucent screen on which ordinary 35 mm slides are projected. In the centre of each slide is a black dot on which Vicki has to fix her gaze. Her distance from the screen is so calculated that the image seen in her right field of view can not be seen in her left field of view, and vice versa. As a result, the picture on the right goes to the left hemisphere, the dominant 'language' side, of the brain, and the picture on the left goes to the right, or usually silent, minor hemisphere of the brain.

The slides show one or two simple line drawings or words, to the left of the dot or to the right. The first slide shows a picture of a football, on the right.

> VICKI: OK, football.
> GAZZANIGA: That's awful fast, give me a chance.

So it is clear that in Vicki's right visual field she sees perfectly well, understands what she sees, and can tell Gazzaniga what she has seen, just as a normal individual would. But when Gazzaniga puts up a slide with the picture to the left of the central dot, the story is rather different. The picture this time is of a girl holding the handset of a telephone and speaking into it.

> GAZZANIGA: Look at the dot.
> VICKI: OK. A woman, a person.
> GAZZANIGA: What else?
> VICKI: A girl, that's all.

But it is clear that Vicki is puzzled. She looks at Gazzaniga questioningly.

> GAZZANIGA: OK, Vicki, I'll tell you what. Open your eyes. I'll put this pencil into your left hand. Now write what she was doing with your left hand. Close your eyes and just let your left hand go.

Vicki closes her eyes and smiles. But as the hand begins to write one can see the letters, ill-formed though they are by her left hand, begin to spell out the word 'telephone'. Gazzaniga takes the paper from her and looks at it. Vicki opens her eyes. Gazzaniga: 'What did you write?' Vicki looks confused and apologetic. She shrugs her shoulders. She doesn't know what she has written on the paper. Gazzaniga questions her again, and this time Vicki answers. 'A skipping rope?' Gazzaniga shows her what she wrote, and Vicki says 'telephone' with some surprise. 'What was she doing?' asks Gazzaniga. 'Talking on the telephone,' says Vicki.

Gazzaniga has developed an interpretation of such events, which explains the functioning of Vicki's separated hemispheres:

> What we saw there was some of the nice interactions of a separate mental system at work. First of all, the right hemisphere apprehended the picture correctly, and said that a woman was being presented to it. However, at the moment that the right hemisphere says 'woman', the left hemisphere hears 'woman' come out of the mouth and it

TESTING VICKI

A) For a split second Vicki was shown a picture of a woman on the phone, so that only her right hemisphere perceived it. She is very unusual in having some language abilities on the right, so could say, 'woman', but no more.
B) The right hemisphere understood more and instructed her left hand to write 'telephone' while her eyes were closed.
C) The left hemisphere was still ignorant about what she had written, and guessed it was 'skipping-rope'.
D) Once shown that she had written the word 'telephone' the left brain knew what the original picture was, as it had already heard the word 'woman'. She then said the picture was of a woman talking on the telephone.

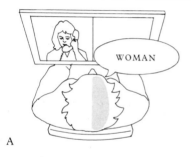

A

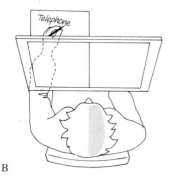

B

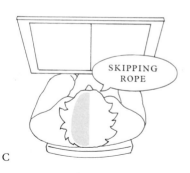

C

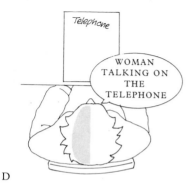

D

now knows that at least part of the stimulus over there involved a woman. And then the left hemisphere begins to try to answer all the questions that I put to Vicki about what the other aspects of the picture were. And, as we saw, she could not expand too much until I asked her to write with her left hand. Now, when Vicki writes with her left hand, which is being controlled by her right hemisphere, it was clear that the right hemisphere had also taken note of the fact there was a telephone in the picture, and was able to write this down. After it had been written, we still pressed Vicki for other aspects, and at this point, the left hemisphere figured out that something must have been going on, so then the left hemisphere began to guess, and made the statement that the woman had something to do with a skipping-rope. Now we know that is the left hemisphere talking, because the right hemisphere (in writing) responded very accurately to what had in fact been in the picture. So what you see in this situation is a right hemisphere with an emerging skill to talk. It captures the correct feature of the picture that there is a woman there, but it doesn't get all of the features. But the writing system of the right hemisphere expressed by the left hand really can capture all of the features, and Vicki is able to write out a full description of what had been presented to the right half brain.

THE HEMISPHERES IN ACTION

Not all the toilers in this particular vineyard would agree with Gazzaniga's interpretation. This may well be because Vicki is unusual: her right hemisphere does seem to be able to talk. In some of Sperry's experiments, 3000 miles away to the west in California, a subject was shown various pictures, selectively to the left and right hemispheres. The right hemisphere was asked, among other things, to make value judgements of portraits of well-known personalities: these were signalled by a 'thumbs up' or a 'thumbs down' gesture. Fidel Castro, Hitler, and a war scene, were among those given a thumbs down response, while thumbs up signals were given for Winston Churchill, Johnny Carson, and pretty girls. (Richard Nixon got a horizontal thumb, whose meaning remains subject to interpretation!) Sperry and his colleagues do not know which spoken comments came from the right hemisphere. They appear to have been limited to short words or comments like 'Wow', 'My God!' and 'Yeah'. Perhaps the most significant fact to emerge during this test was the ability of the right hemisphere to recognize portraits of the experimental subject – that is to say, essentially of itself. (Self-awareness, as shown by a subject's recognition either of his photograph or of himself in a mirror, is taken to have a very close relationship to self-consciousness, and self-consciousness seems to be almost certainly a human quality.) These experiments suggest that, although in most cases the right hemisphere has only limited or even no capacity for speech, nevertheless it is as 'human' as the more verbally gifted left hemisphere. Not everyone, and not even every scientist, would agree. Sir John Eccles, as we have seen, would vehemently disagree.

During Dr Gazzaniga's tests, Vicki gave evidence of the apparent independence of the two halves of her brain. Gazzaniga's apparatus projected a slide which told the left hemisphere to smile and the right hemisphere to clap. Both Vickis did as they were told, but after the experiment the speaking Vicki (the left hemisphere) told us that the only instruction she had seen was the one to smile. Then she began to be a little suspicious.

VICKI: Am I supposed to be seeing two words?
GAZZANIGA: You never can tell. Sometimes yes, sometimes no.

This particular experiment had been arranged so that there was no conflict between the two commands. Had Vicki been asked both to laugh and to frown, it would have been difficult for the two Vickis to react comfortably and the left would probably have dominated. As we found out earlier, the left Vicki and the right Vicki can have quite different ideas about a choice of clothes.

What is the relationship between these two halves of Vicki's brain? We know that the two hemispheres have different skills, as it were, and in particular that language is largely confined to the left hemisphere. Also, the left hemisphere is the dominant hemisphere. But is this simply the situation of one dominant and one submissive partner, or is the relationship somewhat more complex?

Another of Dr Gazzaniga's tests begins to help clear this point up. This time, the familiar projection screen was used, but instead of being asked to speak, Vicki was asked to point with each hand to one of a set of four drawings, the subject of which most closely related to the picture on the screen. Thus, when the pictures were thrown up, the left picture was of an Indian headdress and the right picture was of a submarine. With her right hand, Vicki pointed at a picture of water, and with the left, rather more hesitantly, to a picture of a feather. These indeed were the most closely related subjects available in the four cards near each hand.

GAZZANIGA: Why did you point to those?
VICKI: I pointed to water because it was a boat . . . er . . . (*A long pause here*) . . . Indians. And the boat goes in the water. That's what I've seen.
GAZZANIGA: So what did you see that time?

VICKI: I saw a boat. A boat would float in the water and
on the boat there could be Indians and they would have
feathers. I guess that's all.

Vicki sat back, half smiling, and waited to see how well she had
done. Gazzaniga made cheerful noises.

In some of Dr Sperry's experiments he has suggested the
possibility that the speaking left hemisphere overhears some single
word utterance from the right hemisphere, and guesses at its
significance. So, in the most often quoted example, when the right
hemisphere is shown a picture of a naked person, it is inclined to
provoke a snigger or other symptoms of embarrassment. The
speaking left hemisphere, hearing this, may guess at the content of
the picture which it has not seen. In the test which we have just
quoted, it does not appear that Vicki's left hemisphere could have
picked up enough clues from what it heard to make an adequate
guess. Gazzaniga believes that in Vicki's case, and in some other
cases which he has been studying, there is a rather different
explanation. He believes that the left hemisphere language centre
needs to construct theories about what is going on in the world
which both hemispheres are observing. This need is so intense, he
says, that it seems to be almost impossible to prevent the activity
from going on. He goes on from this to construct a theory about the
whole brain.

> One is trying always to move towards a theory about you
> and me, about what goes into yourself and myself,
> building our sense of subjective reality. And here the
> split brain becomes just a metaphor. It is a situation
> which allows us to make tests, because we know where
> information is in the brain. And we have come to the
> conclusion from studying these patients that we have to
> quit viewing man as a single psychological entity, that in
> fact his psychological self is a multiple self. He has a
> variety of mental systems existing in his brain, most of
> them non-verbal, like the one in his right hemisphere
> tends to be. They have emotions, they have memories,
> they have incentives, they have destinies and they are
> able to control the motor apparatus, to make move-
> ments. They're able to precipitate behaviours on the
> part of someone, and once that action is carried out, the
> left language centre must interpret the action. It must
> give an explanation to itself why the system behaved in
> that way. Why did it just get up and go outside, why did
> it go and order an expensive car when it can't afford it, or
> why did it point at a picture of a feather? Along comes
> this verbal system to give an explanation, and to propose
> a theory to itself. So what we are moving away from is

the idea that there is, in modern parlance, 'a cognitive system', one centre of cognition in the brain. More likely it's a sociological problem, a variety of cognitive centres in the brain all of them being monitored and all of them being closely watched by this dominant language system. This left hemisphere system is trying to maintain consistency and an explanation of all these other systems, and trying to put some sense into their contributions to life's activities.

So to Gazzaniga the left language centres are both master and servant. They sometimes suppress other parts of the brain and sometimes have to explain away embarrassing inconsistent activities controlled by those other parts.

Professor Wall and Sir John Eccles would look at Vicki and her daughter in quite different ways. To Wall, Vicki's responsibility for her daughter Angel emerges from the integrated sensory inputs and movements which are controlled by her now divided brain. But to Eccles, it is only her left hemisphere which causes her to protect her daughter from danger, to feed her and to help educate her. It is in the left hemisphere, Eccles argues, that one may find her mind and her soul.

BLINDSIGHT

We continue to seek enlightenment from the operation of a damaged brain by looking at the case of a young Frenchman. Christian is employed in a workshop for the handicapped in Lyons. At his birth, twenty-five years ago, his left hemisphere was badly damaged by oxygen starvation, which caused severe epilepsy. The remedy was a desperate one. The whole outer section of the left hemisphere of his brain was removed, at the age of seven. Because the operation was performed early in life, it was possible for the language capability to develop in his right hemisphere, so that Christian is able to speak and take part in experiments. At the back of the brain is the visual cortex. The left hemisphere, once again, gives the vision to the right visual field, while the right hemisphere reacts to the left visual field. Remove one hemisphere, containing the visual cortex, and to all intents and purposes the patient is blind on one side. Christian can see only on the left, though, since he can move his head freely, he can shift his point of view to see what he wants and is not unduly handicapped.

What follows is a description of an experiment in which he participated at the Medical Research Institute in Lyons.

The experimental apparatus bears some resemblance to the apparatus Vicki uses. Christian is asked to look straight ahead and his gaze is monitored by a closed-circuit television camera. During the tests, a light is shone on a screen to Christian's left and moved

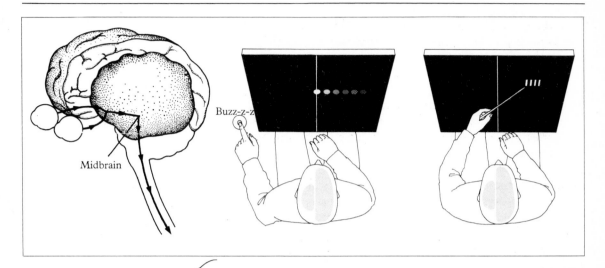

BLINDSIGHT

When given a free choice Christian could not see the light spot on the right until it reached the centre of his field of view (*centre*). He indicated he had seen it by operating the buzzer. He cannot see on the right because of drastic surgery when he was seven years old. Yet when told to point, even if he was not aware of seeing, he pointed correctly (*right*). Asked if he had seen the light bar, he said that he could not, it was luck. So he could see but was unconscious of it!

The explanation for 'blindsight', shown above, involves a pathway in the midbrain which probably does not operate in normally sighted individuals, and in Christian only operates when the conscious control of the upper brain has been relaxed. That is, when he guesses.

gradually towards the centre. He can see it when it is still far to his left, just as a normal individual could. This is his normal extreme angle of view. Next a similar light is shone to his right (his blind side) and moved in again. This time, it cannot be seen until it reaches about the mid-line, just about opposite Christian's nose.

It is important to realize that Christian cannot see the light to his right-hand side when he is asked to report whether he can *see* it. But his reaction to the light changes dramatically when he is no longer asked to report seeing it, but rather to guess its position when the light is at different points close to or far from the centre of his field of view.

The light was flashed momentarily at various locations on Christian's right-hand side. After each brief exposure of the light, he was asked to point with his arm to the direction where he guessed the light might be. After a series of tests, his score stood at between 8 and 9 out of 10. Christian's score was so far above chance that he might almost be described as having vision on a side on which no vision of the normal kind could possibly exist. (And precautions are in operation to guard against the possibility that Christian is glancing to his right.) It is also just possible that, because he was operated on at an early age, some nerve regrowth has taken place which has made connections leading to this strange 'vision'. But the most likely explanation is more straightforward, and based on a number of earlier experiments, both on people and on animals.

All Christian's normal visual pathways on the left were removed, but there is another nerve connection from the eyes into the lower parts of the brain which was not removed. This connects with centres which control arm movements for pointing, and there is a hypothesis that it represents a second visual pathway, which perhaps identifies objects in space and enables an animal (or a man) to direct his gaze at an appropriately interesting part of the world. However, at least in Christian's case, it appears that this pathway only operates under certain conditions, namely when the upper brain permits. That is to say, when Christian is prepared to guess rather than to make a definite, conscious choice of the position of the light. Christian's surprising visual ability, then, can be explained entirely on the basis of brain structure. It is only when the unconscious part of the brain is left to its own devices that the phenomenon occurs, and it does not appear to be necessary to invoke the entity of the mind to explain it. Indeed, when the mind may be taken to be in operation, the phenomenon disappears.

Such evidence from people whose brain structure is so manifestly abnormal can scarcely be conclusive. But it is possible to examine a rather similar phenomenon in a 'normal' individual, where the evidence is perhaps easier to evaluate.

HEARING WITHOUT LISTENING

Our 'normal' individual is Professor Daniel Dennett, the philosopher from Tufts University in Boston, who agreed to take part in an experiment devised by Dr J R Lackner from the nearby Brandeis University. A tape recorder is used to play two different sentences, one to each ear of the experimental subject. The subject is told to attend to one ear only, and to paraphrase the sentence he hears in that ear. A sentence is played to the 'attended' ear, whose construction makes it ambiguous. For example, 'The corrupt police can't stop drinking.' The other ear hears, slightly later and at a lower volume, a sentence which elucidates the ambiguous sentence, which in the case of the corrupt police might be, 'The cops were drunk again.'

Professor Dennett listened to a series of tests, and paraphrased what he heard. One of the sentences played into the ear to which he was instructed to attend was 'Visiting relatives can be a bore'. Into the other ear, at lower volume, the sentence 'I don't like to visit relatives' was played. Professor Dennett reported his reactions:

> Going to visit my relatives is a bore. Now what I might
> have said is, I can't stand it when my relatives show up,
> but that's not what I said, and the reading I came up with
> is in fact the one suggested by what was coming in on my
> right ear, as I later learned. At the time I was utterly
> oblivious of what was coming in on my right ear.

Professor Dennett devotes much of his time to consideration of the mind/brain problem, and he regards this experiment as being of considerable importance.

> What this experiment shows very graphically is that
> quite outside our consciousness our minds are engaged

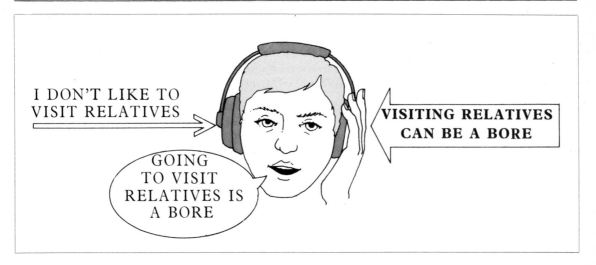

UNCONSCIOUS UNDERSTANDING

The person being tested listens with his left ear to a sentence which may have at least two interpretations, and tries to paraphrase it. *At the same time* a second sentence is played into his right ear which could clarify the ambivalent sentence. In most cases the subject's response has been influenced by the right ear's sentence, even though he was not conscious of hearing it. This means that the brain can analyze and comprehend language unconsciously as well as consciously.

in elaborate and sophisticated activity, analysing incoming signals, leading eventually to comprehension of the meanings not just of the words but of the sentences heard. Experiments of this sort have led to something of a revolution in our understanding of the mind. It used to be thought that the mind seemed to be transparent to itself. The method of introspection ideally revealed to each individual person the total contents and activities of his mind; the very idea of unconscious mental activity was viewed as something of a contradiction. Now it looks almost the other way round, as we reveal more and more of the unconscious mental activity that contributes to the control of our bodies. The part that is conscious begins to look like the tip of the iceberg, and as we begin to develop sketchy models of how the brain, and only the brain, can operate to account for the unconscious mental activity, the prospect emerges of being able to explain the conscious part as well with a set of hypotheses which involve nothing but statements about the operation of the nerves and nerve cells in the brain.

It was Professor Dennett who invented the science fiction situation mentioned at the beginning of this chapter: the story of the disembodied brain. How might he feel if it happened to him, if it was his brain he was standing looking at?

Of course, part of my imaginary self's impressions come from the actual position of my eyes in my body, my point of view. In addition though, that point of view is constructed from all the memories, habits and so forth stored in my brain, and its mental activities now that it's under its glass dome. But since these mental activities depend on input from the senses in my body and can be expressed only through my body, they seem to be in my body.

So this sense of 'I' myself is not a mysterious pearl of mind-stuff, nor is it a little hunk of brain tissue. It's an abstraction. Some abstract objects can be located in space and time – the equator for instance, or the centre of gravity of a table lamp. But an abstraction like 'myself' is more difficult to locate because it is the sum of all the activities of my body. 'Myself' is created by my body and brain acting together.

What Professor Dennett describes as his 'thought experiment' is, of course, a more extreme version of the sort of operation that was in fact performed on Vicki, our friend with the split brain. And Professor Dennett had comments to make on Vicki's case.

As long as one half of Vicki's brain isn't being isolated from the other and information goes into both halves, she is only one person in one body. But if we carefully arrange an isolation between the halves, so that slightly different and conflicting information, intentions, activities can develop in each hemisphere, then we're led irresistibly to the idea of two selves – the Vicki that goes with the left and the Vicki that goes with the right.

SCIENCE AND RELIGION

Words can be a barrier to understanding. All of us place slightly different constructions, no doubt, on the words 'mind', 'consciousness' and 'self'. Philosophers and psychologists give each their own meanings, more precise than the layman. But for most of us the three words put together amount to one idea, as we intimated at the beginning of this chapter, and for that idea the Christian thinker might substitute another word, 'soul'.

If, like Sir John Eccles, you are a Christian, then there is no question that the soul, or the mind, or the self, exists, nor that it is a non-physical, non-material thing. 'Yes, I do believe in the supernatural,' says Eccles.

I do believe that we are the product of the creativity of what we call God. I hope that this life will lead to some future existence where my self or soul will have another existence, with another brain, or computer if you like. I don't know how I got this one, it's a pretty good one, and I'm very grateful for it, but I do know as a realist that it will disappear and with it all my detailed memories. But I think my conscious self or soul will come through.

Most scientists, and all materialists, would disagree with him. But there are plenty of other scientists who echo Sir John's religious conviction. It may be arrogant for either side in the argument to believe that the opposite view is totally untenable, but at the moment it seems to come down to a matter of faith, either in a supernatural world or in scientific evidence. The pieces of evidence offered by the world of science are less directly understood than we might like, but at least they point to some of the amazing capabilities of the brain. It seems that the brain can process many channels of information simultaneously. It seems, too, that many of those channels are being processed below the level we call consciousness, through emotional centres and those which are responsible for movement and other more automated functions of the human being, but also in part, as Professor Dennett's listening experiment shows, through language centres too. Perhaps all these processes are supervised, and made sense of, by the language capability in the left half of the brain, which then proceeds to explain the actions of the whole human being not only to the world but to itself.

For thousands of years, philosophers have puzzled their brains far into the night to attempt to understand what those brains are doing, and how it can be described. For the last two hundred years or so, the period of the scientific study of the brain, scientists, too, have been puzzled. There have never been more scientists working on the subject of the brain than there are today, and many of them are now as anxious as the philosophers to understand its functioning as a whole. Of all the questions, the most intractable is the riddle of what the mind is, and where it might be found. As we have seen, it is possible to experiment, albeit in very special circumstances, with the brain and to gain at least some inkling of what mind might be. If the mind is, as Professors Wall and Dennett think, a process of the brain and body, then our understanding of the brain may lead to an understanding of the mind, and of the self. If we can gain that understanding, it will be the most important of all the discoveries of science.

THE NEXT FIFTY YEARS

Predictions almost always prove to be wrong, even in the short term. Perhaps their only lasting value is to provide innocent amusement for future readers. But it is impossible to hold conversations with scientists on the topic of the human brain without picking up some sense of the uncertain future. The scientists themselves are rightly and understandably cautious of speculation. Where they speculate about areas which may be the subject of clinical work with patients, they are careful not to raise hopes for the future; it may be better for the patient to suffer in ignorance than to be offered hope that may turn out to be cruelly false. Where, in the preceding pages, scientists have guessed at the future, they have been careful to label their statements so that they may not be mistaken for objective truth, if that can be said to exist at all. So any predictions made here are not to be attributed to any of the scientists whose work we have discussed. But they all have some basis in evidence that has been presented to us.

Vicki, the split-brain patient in our previous chapter, was treated for severe and intractable epilepsy by what is usually described as 'heroic' surgery. It is not possible to conclude that her surgery was a mistake, because though she still has major (*grand mal*) seizures they are not as frequent as they were before the operation. However, that operation is not done in Britain and is clearly one that only a few surgeons in the United States are willing to do. It therefore comes into the category in which one hopes there will be the greatest improvement in the next decades: radical treatments undertaken because there is nothing else to be done. If the accumulation of information about the brain achieves nothing else it should improve the sophistication of medical treatment. Until now that has often been unavoidably crude and has included, for example, electro-convulsive therapy, removal of parts of the brain (already much less frequent), and insulin shock treatment for schizophrenia. Today, much promise is held out for more accurate diagnosis and localization of brain damage. The CAT scan and the PET scan which we encountered in Chapter 2 are such new tools that for the first time neurologists can see what areas are damaged without subjecting the patient to surgery. Other similar techniques are emerging all the time, which means that surgery, too, when it is needed, may be more localized and therefore less damaging – lasers are already available for this task. Less dramatic, but in its way equally impressive, is the extensive use of drugs like Valium and Librium for treatment of anxiety. Some forms of anxiety might be treatable by discussion and therapy, as spider phobia is, others by more precise use of better drugs when they become available. The greatest improvement might be a social one: the acceptance by the medical profession that human neuroses are best treated by human contact; possibly with the help of drugs, but not by the indiscriminate prescription of drugs alone. Our knowledge of the brain is showing more and more clearly that we can sometimes influence its chemistry and its internal workings as effectively by psychological means as by such external influences as drugs or operations. So the first step forward in the next decades might be a general one: the more human treatment of brain disorders at each end of the spectrum of severity – from anxiety to madness. Such a step would involve committing more staff to the treatment of mental illness, and testing society's will to invest more in psychiatric care.

In our chapter on fear we mentioned – and our parachutist example demonstrated – how that emotion, when stimulated, could affect learning, and affect it by means of the brain's chemical actions. As so much research into emotions is now concentrating on brain chemicals one immediately thinks that such research could lead to 'learning pills', which would contain the chemicals that influence emotions and improve learning. However, such developments may well be impractical. No drugs are known which do not have side-effects and therefore there must be a balance between benefits and deficits. But though learning drugs may be unlikely, we should be able to improve learning by discovering what emotional states improve it most, and encouraging them in the student. If we choose the right emotions, it may not only improve learning but make it a more pleasant experience as well!

The processing of language in the brain is not by any means understood, yet it is just becoming possible to get computers to understand very simple stories in the way humans do. At Yale University a computer has been programmed to respond in a very human way to a story about a teacher, John, who goes into a restaurant, has some trouble with the waitress and leaves without paying his bill. Simple though the story is, in order to answer questions about why John was upset the computer requires a great deal of knowledge: about restaurants, what one expects of waitresses, that one has to pay bills to them and so on. To give the computer this information turned out to be a mammoth programming task, but its success shows that in the future computers may well take over some human language functions. At first this will probably be, for example, answering telephone enquiries about train and plane timetables. The technology will soon be available to convert simple spoken requests into a form computers can use; and the reverse, technology to convert their output back into speech, already exists. It could be an unnerving experience if one does not know whether the voice at the other end is a human or a computer; but the language capability of computers seems a very long way from anything more sophisticated than answering timetable requests so far.

The other possibility in the area of language is to be able to give much needed help for stroke victims. As Charles Landry shows, recovery from a stroke can take place, depending on the individual and his damage, but we are only just beginning to try ways of improving it or speeding it up. In Professor Geschwind's unit in Boston, Dr Nancy Helm has been trying to use musical rhythms. The theory is based on the observation that many stroke patients with virtually no language can still sing, and use words in singing which they never use in speech. This is because melody is associated with the undamaged right hemisphere. In the United States and in some centres in England, Dr Helm is training patients by getting them to speak to a simple rhythm. It helps some patients, and therapists hope it will lead to improved methods for the future; as the numbers suffering from language disorders runs into tens of thousands even in Britain, better methods are urgently needed.

Far more people are handicapped by the immense range of disorders of movement. Some of them will undoubtedly be treatable by drugs (like the L-DOPA that Terry Thomas takes now), but the as yet undeveloped techniques of brain transplants may turn out to be more useful. If young rats can be given transplants of the cells that make dopamine, perhaps humans can too. Perhaps other types of cells can be transplanted to treat other diseases caused by low levels of brain chemicals: schizophrenia is one obvious example. Since in some cases it is the general level of a chemical that is too low, the transplanted cells may not have to grow at a specific place in the brain.

There are signs that a simpler treatment will be used for a whole range of disorders: eating. Already some preliminary evidence has led to the suggestion that old people will become senile less quickly, or even have their brain function improved, by eating more lecithin (a constituent of some fats). Lecithin is the raw material of choline, and choline is an important constituent of the nerve cells whose death seems to cause senile dementia. No one yet knows for sure whether the treatment works, but it is one example of research into diet and the brain which may lead to improvements in the treatment of everything from Parkinson's Disease to recovery from strokes or anxiety.

It is no accident that research into vision at the Massachusetts Institute of Technology is supported by grants from the US Defence Department. An artificial eye and brain, or even the first stages of it, would be a great boon to any country's armed forces.

Surveillance systems would no longer need human eyes. Rocket guidance systems could possibly be based on what there was to see of the target rather than on infra-red radiation or any other signals from the target. In the next decades there will undoubtedly also be the beginnings of artificial eyes and computer brains for peaceful uses. Artificial limbs, too, will eventually be improved by work on the control of movement in the nervous system.

The outstanding development in the next few decades will almost certainly be the production of new drugs for the brain. Despite governmental controls on the introduction of new drugs, pharmaceutical companies still flourish and the fast expanding knowledge of brain chemistry will continue to be utilized by them. For example, work on Valium and Librium receptors shows that these drugs may have specific effects in different areas of the brain and there will probably be a new wave of chemicals for treating different types of anxiety. However, the immense effort channelled into that research might be better (if less profitably) spent in investigating, improving and promoting alternative treatments based on behaviour therapy, like that used for Beverley and her spider phobia. All drugs have unexpected side-effects and need to be used cautiously.

Brain chemistry is fast throwing up fascinating connections between the brain and the body. Some brain chemicals are also found in the intestines. This apparently bizarre connection is not so surprising, because brain and gut are closely connected in the early life of the developing foetus. If the functions of chemicals in each place are connected, this research may eventually lead to a clearer understanding of psychosomatic illness. Chemicals from the brain undoubtedly affect the body in ways we do not yet understand. They often trigger the production of other chemicals which in turn affect the brain. This area of knowledge may well help us to cope with our feelings and understand what is going on when we get angry, fall in love, or appreciate music.

One major discovery during the last few years of research in brain chemistry is that of the endorphins: the 'morphines' produced by the brain itself. These chemicals are released by the brain under numerous circumstances, from acupuncture to jogging and cocktail parties, and we will undoubtedly find how to manipulate their levels more and more effectively as knowledge about them grows. We may be able to develop non-addictive pain-killers, based on the structure of the endorphins; though early promise here has not yet been fulfilled.

Although brain chemistry is at present a growth area, there may soon be a subtle change of direction. Many chemicals act at the synapse, and thereby control the passage of nerve signals very effectively, but there are some electrical synapses, not controlled by chemicals, which are not well described, but offer the possibility of a completely new field of research. Already electrical stimulation or suppression is used to treat otherwise intractable pain and paralysis, with some effect. It could be that such treatments will enter a new era in which they become alternatives to drugs.

So much of our knowledge about the brain is piecemeal and is so detailed that it is difficult to generalize from it to the human being. The analogy of a computer is a useful one, and it will become more so, but since it now seems that nerve cells may be subtly more than simple on/off switches, that analogy may have to be modified. It could be that the wheel will turn full circle and our knowledge of the brain will lead to new types of computer.

No discovery is without its dangers. Unscrupulous individuals may well misuse the discoveries of psychologists or neuro-scientists, and it is impossible to provide secure safeguards against this contingency. But it is more dangerous to turn against the investigators and trust instead to mysticism, ignorance and fantasy. If the quest is for relevance, there are few more relevant studies for the human brain *than* the human brain: and we are only just at the beginning of that great journey of discovery. As the glare of research turns to one area and then another, knowledge ebbs and flows. In the future, some of our dogmas may be disproved. Perhaps the synapse may not be so central a feature of brain function as we now think; perhaps the cerebral cortex may be dethroned from its position as the most characteristically 'human' part of the brain. Science will certainly lead in many unexpected directions; as long as we remember that our brains are important because they make us human, not because they are so complicated and interesting, these studies will help us grow in humanity and not merely in knowledge.

GLOSSARY

ADRENALIN A hormone secreted by the adrenal glands. There is some evidence also that it is used as a NEUROTRANSMITTER.

ALEXIA The inability to read, often caused by damage to the language areas of the brain.

ANXIETY A rather generalized term which covers clinical states varying from fear of a particular situation or object to so-called 'free floating anxiety' which has no special object. There is some controversy over its precise meaning.

APHASIA Impaired language caused by a STROKE, or any other damage to the brain. The patient makes errors in either word order or word choice or both, not just in pronunciation.

AXON The output fibre of a nerve cell (or NEURONE), usually carrying signals to other cells. In some exceptional cases it may receive input.

BLOCKERS Drugs whose action is to block cell RECEPTORS by occupying them and thereby prevent the action of a hormone or neurotransmitter, for example.

BRAIN SLICE In the technique of 'brain slice' physiology a thin slice, usually of some regularly arranged region, especially cerebellum or hippocampus, can be kept working for up to 24 hours in a suitable fluid and used for experiments.

CELL REGENERATION Dead brain cells are not replaced, but the fibres of some damaged cells may grow again through this process.

DENDRITE The fibre of the nerve cell which usually serves to receive signals; usually it is many-branched.

DYSLEXIA Impaired reading, often associated with children.

ECT Electro Convulsive Therapy. This is an electric shock applied to the brain while the patient is anaesthetized. It is used mainly as an attempt to treat severe depression. Although this method has been very widely used, it is increasingly falling into disfavour.

HABITUATION The process by which a nerve cell adapts to a stimulus and ceases to send signals in response to it.

HALLUCINATION Seeing, hearing, touching, smelling or tasting a sensation which does not actually exist.

HYPNOSIS Putting someone willingly into a trance-like state in which they will accept suggestions from the hypnotist.

ILLUSION An optical illusion is a pattern which fools the eye and brain in some way. For example, it may appear lighter, or longer than it really is.

MADNESS A state in which an individual's thought and reason are sufficiently abnormal and disordered that he or she cannot effectively communicate, in the broadest sense, with others and so cannot function in society.

MNEMONIC A device, usually verbal, to aid memory: e.g. "Thirty days hath September".

NERVE CELL See NEURONE.

NEURONE A nerve cell, including all its fibres. It may be in the brain, the spinal cord, or the peripheral nervous system.

NEUROTRANSMITTER A substance released at synapses which relays a nerve signal from one nerve cell to others. They include noradrenalin, dopamine, serotonin and acetylcholine.

PEPTIDES A class of substances made up of short chains of amino-acids, joined end to end. Some neurotransmitters are thought to be peptides.

PHOBIA An extreme fear, usually morbid and often irrational.

PLETHYSMOGRAPH A device for measuring the volume of blood in the blood vessels.

PSYCHOSIS Mental illness so severe that the individual's personality is destroyed and he or she cannot function normally.

RECEPTOR There are receptors throughout the body. The nerve cell is shaped to receive chemical molecules, thus causing a response in the cell. Other kinds of receptors include light receptors in the retina and heat receptors in the skin.

SCHIZOPHRENIA A group of mental illnesses causing madness. Thoughts and feelings are not connected with each other and either or both of them may be disordered.

SENSITIZATION In general the opposite of HABITUATION. A sensitized cell will respond more readily to a stimulus.

STEREOGRAM Two pictures, each viewed by one eye, which when combined by the brain give the illusion of a three-dimensional shape.

STRESS Like ANXIETY a rather generalized term. The pressure of work, for example, may be a stress which leads to an exaggerated state of anxiety which needs treatment.

SYNAPSE The region where nerve cells communicate, usually by means of NEUROTRANSMITTERS.

STROKE Brain damage caused by a blocked or burst blood vessel. Tissue round the blood vessel may die from starvation due to either lack of blood, or swelling.

SYNTAX The grammatical arrangement of words in either speech or writing.

TOMOGRAPHY 'Slice-writing'. A technique, exemplified by the CAT scan (Computerized Axial Tomography) in which successive 'slices' of the brain are viewed by X-ray or some other means, and the information processed to yield a picture of the internal structure of the brain, with a view to locating regions of injury or disease.

VESICLE A small globule or bag. Synaptic vesicles, for example, are tiny bags of membrane which contain the neurotransmitter substance inside the nerve cell or neurone.

FURTHER READING

A vast amount of highly specialist literature exists on the human brain. This list of suggested books is not meant to be an exhaustive bibliography, but to give the interested layman some useful pointers to exploring the subject further.

Alan D. Baddeley, *The Psychology of Memory*, Harper & Row, New York 1976
A clear account of its subject which helpfully does not conceal the arguments and ambiguities inherent in it.

Calder, Nigel, *The Mind of Man*, BBC Publications, London 1970
An intriguing account, lucidly expressed and well illustrated, of the state of the science in the previous decade. By no means of only historical interest.

Cooper, Jack R., *The Biochemical Basis of Neuropharmacology*, Oxford University Press, New York 1978
A very detailed but straightforward account of brain chemistry, frank in its admission of our ignorance, and entertainingly written.

Cotman, Carl W., and McGaugh, James L., *Behavioural Neuroscience*, Academic Press Inc., New York 1980
Probably the best single account of modern theories linking the brain to human behaviour. Clearly written and lavishly, if not always stylishly, illustrated.

Dennett, Daniel, *Brainstorms*, Harvester Press, Brighton 1981
A series of essays on the problems of the brain and mind by a philosopher who is unusually easy to understand.

Geschwind, Norman, and Reidel, D., *Selected Papers on Language and the Brain*, D. Reidel Publishing Co., Boston, Mass. 1974
Geschwind is an entertaining and informative writer, whose passion for his subject is well conveyed.

Granit, Ragnar, *The Purposive Brain*, MIT Press, Cambridge, Mass. 1977
An account by the doyen of Swedish neurologists of his theory of voluntary movement. Stimulating if occasionally obscure.

Hofstadter, Douglas R., and Dennett, Daniel, *The Mind's I*, Harvester Press, Brighton 1981
A follow-up to *Brainstorms*.

Kandel, Eric R., *Cellular Basis of Behaviour: An Introduction to Behavioural Neurobiology*, W.H. Freeman and Co., San Francisco 1976
Kandel has sometimes been criticized for a reductionist approach, but he combines rigorous science with keen insights into human behaviour, and is outstanding in his field.

Kelly, Desmond, *Anxiety and Emotions*, Charles C. Thomas, Springfield, Illinois 1980
A readable account by an author whose contact with patients illuminates his more general points.

Liddell, E. G. T., *The Discovery of Reflexes*, Oxford University Press, Oxford 1960
A stimulating account with excellent illustrations of the early history of neuroscience.

Luria, A. R., *The Mind of a Mnemonist* (translated from the Russian by L. Solotaroff), Jonathan Cape, London 1969
Fascinating account of the tragedy of a man who could not forget.

Marr, David, *Seeing: a Computational Approach*, W.H. Freeman and Co., San Francisco 1982
A major new approach to human vision. Hard-going, but very clearly and logically written and well worth the effort. The conversation at the end is very helpful.

Phillips, C. G., and Porter, R., *Corticospinal Neurones: Their Role in Movement*, Academic Press Inc., New York 1977
Despite its gloomy title, an entertaining account of current thoughts on brain systems for movement control; a precise and balanced view.

Rose, Steven, *The Conscious Brain*, Random House, New York 1976
A clear account for the layman, well written and aptly illustrated. The author's political views only occasionally intrude.

Sherrington, Sir Charles, *The Integrative Activity of the Nervous System*, Arno Press 1973, Cambridge University Press, Cambridge 1947
The indispensable and classic account of the nervous system. Some facts are now challengeable, but Sherrington's ideas are always stimulating and sometimes inspiring.

Smythies, John R. (ed.) *Brain and Mind*, Routledge, London 1979
A collection from a CIBA symposium with views from experts on consciousness in many fields. Very thought-provoking.

Snyder, Solomon H., *Madness and the Brain*, McGraw-Hill Inc., New York 1974
Although this book is some years old it is a very clear account of the relationship between schizophrenia and the brain by a leading researcher in the field.

Warwick, Roger, and Williams, Peter L. (eds.), *Gray's Anatomy*, 36th edition, Churchill Livingstone, Edinburgh, London, Melbourne and New York 1980
The section on neurology is finely illustrated, and an admirable introduction to the basic features of the brain and nervous system.

de Wied, D., and van Keep, P.A. (eds.), *Hormones and the Brain*, MIT Press, Cambridge, Mass. 1980
A collection of papers on one of the fastest-growing areas of neuroscience.

Young, J. Z., *Programs of the Brain*, Oxford University Press, Oxford 1978
A thoroughly entertaining and sometimes challenging general account by Britain's most respected neuroscientist, looking back over a lifetime of experiment and discovery.

Index

Picture Acknowledgments

PHOTOGRAPHS
The publishers would like to acknowledge the picture sources listed below and thank them for their invaluable contribution to this book.
Dr Floyd E Bloom, Salk Institute California page 107, 126;
Dr Anders Bjorklund, University of Lund page 107;
Bridgeman Art Library page 80, 159;
BBC page 10, 11, 46, 54, 127;
BBC/Mat Irvine page 163;
British Leyland page 103;
Dr M J and MRs F A Burton, Scientific Photography page 19, 20, 106;
Camera Press page 141, 153;
Musée Dupuytren, Paris page 50;
Musée Dupuytren, Paris/Jean Loup Charmet page 53;
Dr Gary Lynch, micrograph retouched by Roy Flooks page 41;
Susannah Fiennes page 77;
Gordon G Gallup Jr, State University New York page 134;
Goethe Museum, Frankfurt page 159;
Dr Miles Herkenham/Dr Candace Pert, National Institute of Mental Health, Bethesda, Maryland page 108, 125;
Professor T Hokfelt, Karolinska Institute, Stockholm page 126;
R C James page 94;
Richard Jameson page 149t, 150;
David Johnson page 1, 10, 11, 29, 35, 39, 49, 51, 154, 168, 171;
Dr R Llinas, University of New York Medical School page 105, 114, 116;
Dr Margaret A Naeser Ph.D, Aphasia Research Center Department of Neurology. Boston University School of Medicine and Boston Veterans Administrative Medical Center. CT scan from Radiology Service Dr Harvey Levine, Boston Veterans Administration Medical Center page 49;
Oxford Mail 14th May 1960 page 149b;
Popperphoto page 141, 142;
Rex Features page 141;

Rowan Gallery, London page 88;
Salvador Dali Museum, St Petersburg Florida/SPADEM page 87;
Sunday Times page 2, 61;
Justine Todd illustration commissioned for *Centre of the Cyclone* by John C Lilly published by courtesy of Granada Publishing page 160;
John Topham Library page 141;
UPI page 15;
Max Whitby page 54, 60, 89, 131;
Whitney Museum of American Art, New York. Tempera on composition board 18 × 36, Juliana Force purchase page 159;

ARTWORK
The Publishers would like to thank those who provided the artwork references listed below, and also Dee McLean and Clive Spong of Linden Artists, and David Johnson who in many cases adapted these references for the purposes of this book.
Stephen Hopkinson page 76;
David Johnson page 18 from *Psychology of Memory* by Alan Baddeley. Copyright © 1976 by Basic Books Inc. By permission of Basic Books, Inc., Publishers, New York.
Page 32, page 56 adapted from *Scientific American* September 1979 Volume 241 No 3 'Specializations of the Human Brain' by Norman Geschwind page 163; page 94, 127, 131, 141, 142, 146, 153 adapted from *Schizophrenia* paper © Office Health Economics;
Dee McLean page 12, 13, 25 drawing Eric Kandel's paper *Harvey Lectures series 73* © 1979 Academic Press; page 49, 67, 70, 71, 76, 82 adapted from *Seeing* by John P Frisby Oxford University Press © 1979 figure 62 after C Blakemore (1973) *The Baffled Brain.* In R L Gregory and E H Gombrich (1973) *Illusion in Art and Nature* Duckworth; page 109 adapted from *Scientific American* 1979: 'Brain Mechanisms of Movement' by Edward V Evarts page 154; page 111 taken

from *Integrative Action of the Nervous System* by Sherrington, Cambridge University Press; page 112 adapted from *Scientific American* May 1972 page 35 of 'How we control the Contraction of our Muscles' by P A Merton; page 114, page 129 adapted from *Introduction to Psychology* 7th edition by Ernest R Hilgart © 1979 Harcourt Brace Jovanovich by permission of the publishers; 138–139, 156, 165, 177b
Richard E M Moore © page 105 published in *Gray's Anatomy* 36th edition Churchill Livingston © Longman Group Limited page 920 figure 7.79 redrawn from *The Cerebellum as a Neuronal Machine* by J C Eccles, M Ito and J Szentagothai Springer 1967.
A Pellionisz and R Llinas drawing taken from their paper published in *Neuroscience* Volume 4 page 341 1979 Pergamon Press London page 116;
Scientific American June 1974 page 62 'Neurotransmitters' by Julius Axelrod page 120;
Clive Spong page 12, 21, 35 adapted from the Pegword System from *The Brain Book* page 126 by Peter Russell Routledge & Kegan Paul; page 74, 90–92 in conjunction with material published by David Marr and H Keith Nishihara *Technology Review* Volume 81 Number 1 October 1978 © 1978 Alumni Association of the Massachusetts Institute of Technology, Cambridge; page 99 adapted from *Children and Exercise IX* edited by K Berg and B O Erikkson © 1980 page 34–35 University Park Press; page 104, page 137 based on material supplied by Dr Raja Ghosh; page 169 adapted from *Scientific American* August 1967 page 28 top of 'The Split Brain in Man' by Michael S Gazzaniga; page 173 adapted from R W Sperry paper published in *Neuropsychologia 9* 1971 Neurological Institute New York; page 177, 179.